MOCKTAIL
Hour

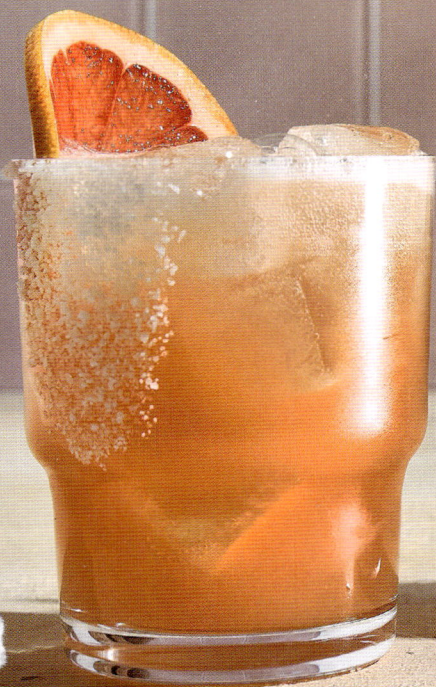

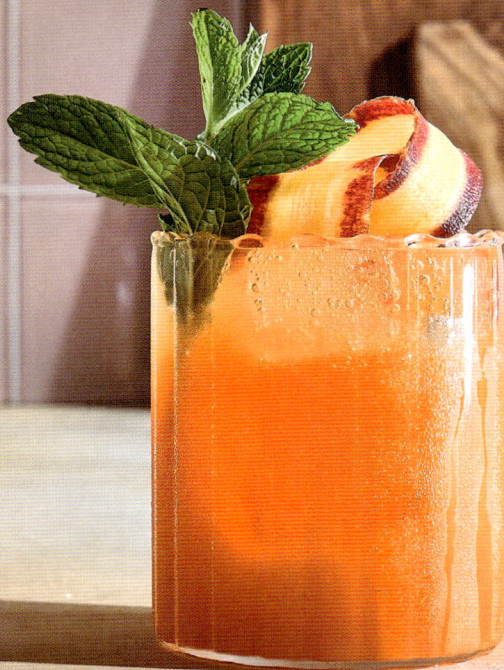

70 Sips for Anytime Delights
and Hangover-Free Nights

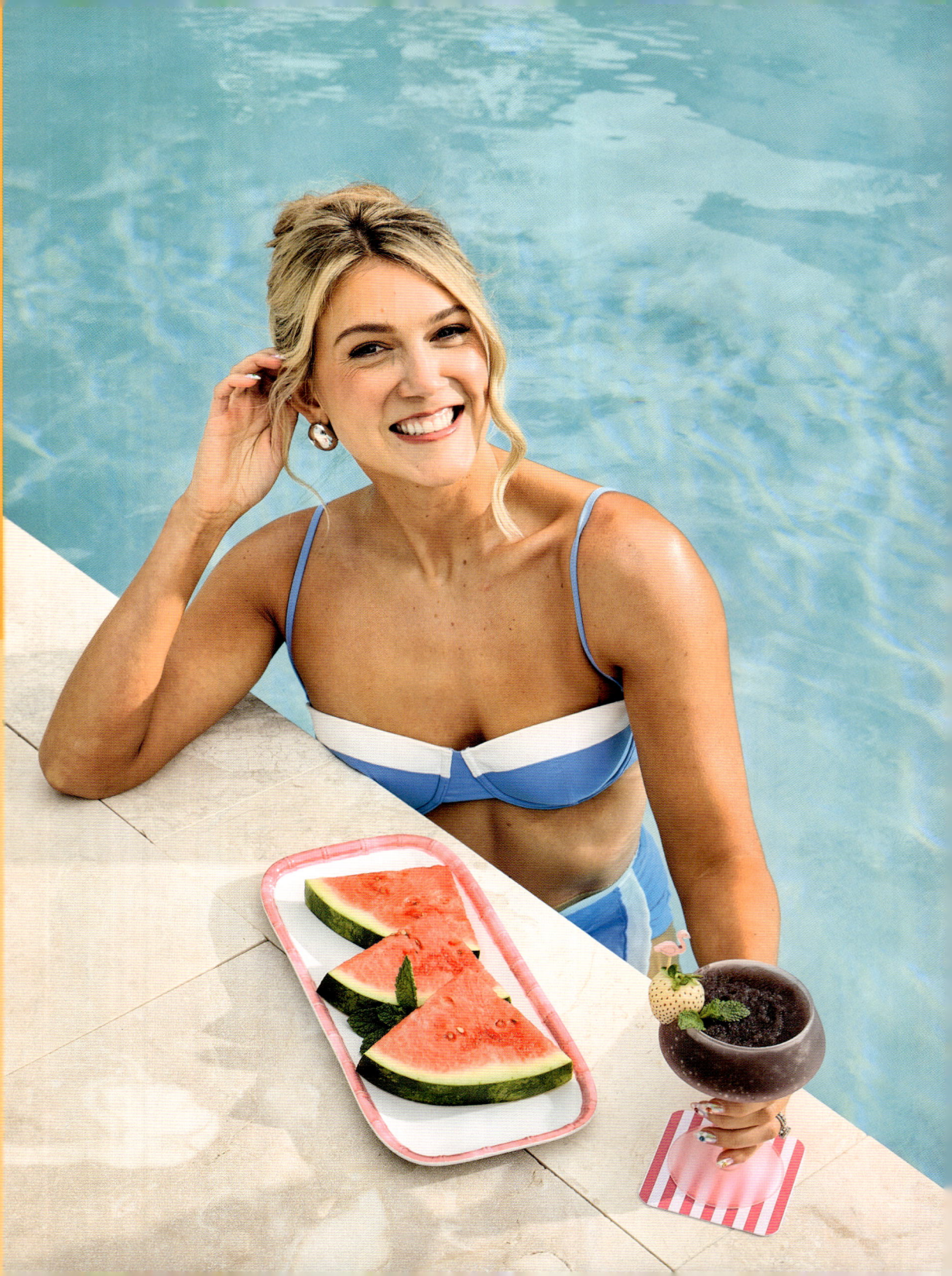

callie gullickson

MOCKTAIL
Hour

70 Sips for Anytime Delights and
Hangover-Free Nights

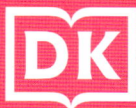

DK

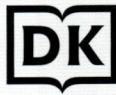

DK | Penguin Random House

Publisher Mike Sanders
Art & Design Director William Thomas
Editorial Director Ann Barton
Executive Editor Olivia Peluso
Editorial Assistant Resham Anand
Designer Amy Sly, The Sly Studio
Page Layout Maluhia Nahuina, The Sly Studio
Photographer Ashleigh Amoroso

Drink Stylists Maite Aizpurua & Kristina Kitchen
Prop Stylists Audrey Davis & Kristina Kitchen
Digital Tech Javier Sanchez
Photography Assistants Hannah Casparian, Ish Holmes & Leigh Skomal
Copyeditor Mira S. Park
Proofreaders Taylor Plett & Bianca Bosman
Indexer Louisa Emmons

First American Edition, 2025
Published in the United States by DK Publishing
1745 Broadway, 20th Floor, New York, NY 10019

The authorized representative in the EEA is Dorling Kindersley
Verlag GmbH. Arnulfstr. 124, 80636 Munich, Germany

A catalog record for this book is available from the Library of Congress.
ISBN 978-0-5939-5865-0

DK books are available at special discounts when purchased
in bulk for sales promotions, premiums, fund-raising, or
educational use. For details, contact SpecialSales@dk.com

Printed and bound in China
www.dk.com

MIX
Paper | Supporting
responsible forestry
FSC™ C018179

This book was made with Forest
Stewardship Council™ certified
paper – one small step in DK's
commitment to a sustainable future.
Learn more at
www.dk.com/uk/information/sustainability

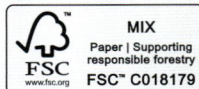

Dedication

To those who confidently embrace their individuality, and to everyone who makes time for self-care moments. May each sip empower you and remind you of the strength in prioritizing yourself.

Mocktail Hour CONTENTS

ENERGY ELIXIRS

MOOD BOOSTERS

SELF-CARE SIPS

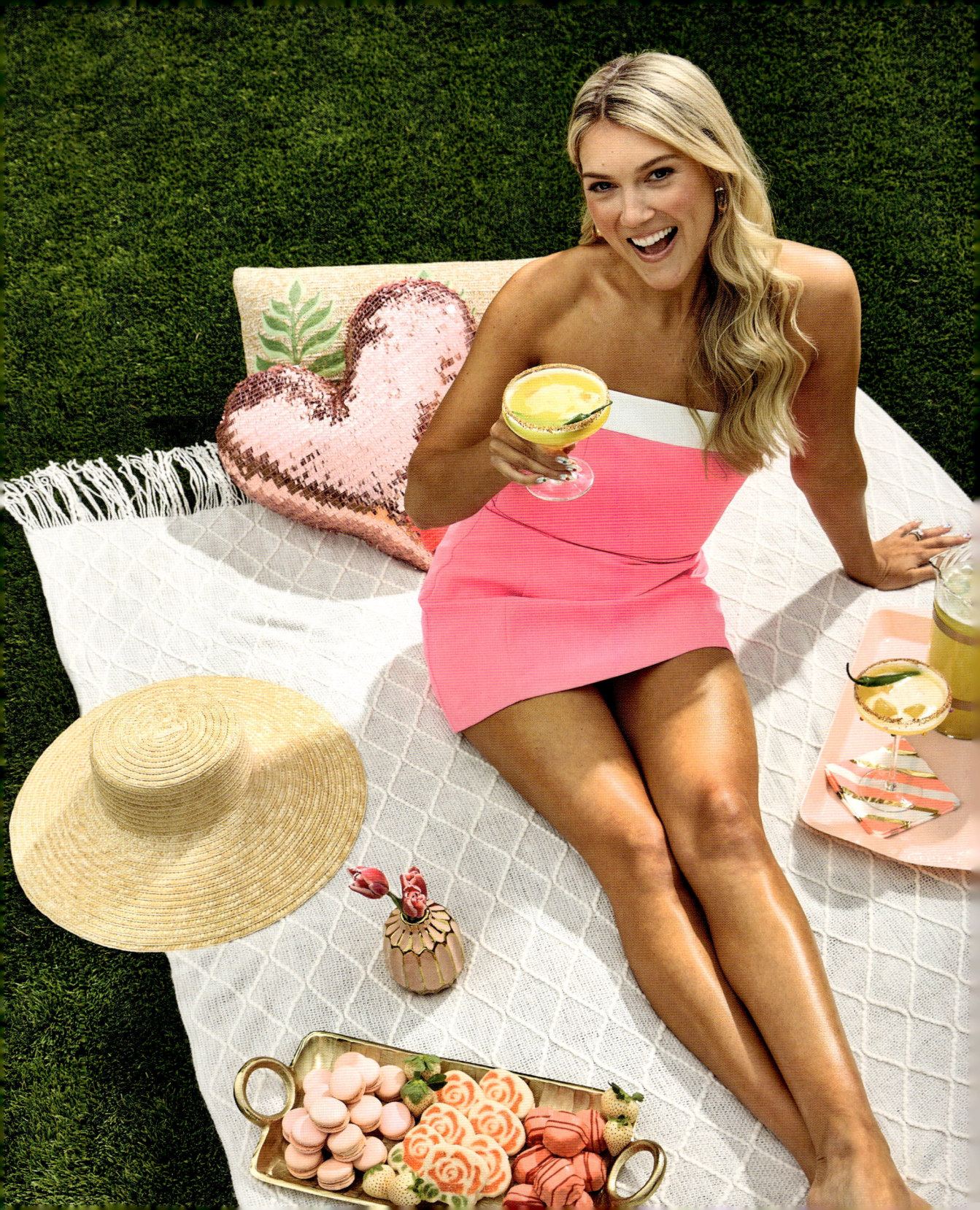

INTRODUCTION

Hey, besties! It's time to show ourselves some self-care without sacrificing on the fun. Let's be honest: Having fun shouldn't come at the price of not feeling our best. Which is why it's time to introduce you to *Mocktail Hour*—that hour of each day when you can sip, shake, and say yes to feeling fabulous. I am here to share some seriously delicious mocktail recipes that will add a dash of fun and flavor to your everyday life. Whether you're taking a break from booze, looking for refreshing alternatives, or just want to mix things up, *Mocktail Hour* has got your back. When I say no fancy bartending skills are required, I mean it!

Why do I need this book, Callie? Glad you asked. I believe we work way too hard to feel good physically and mentally on a day-to-day basis just to throw it all away after a few drinks. Sure, drinking alcohol may feel good in the moment, but the next morning (or the next three days, if you're like me) we all ask ourselves the same question: "Why did I do that?" Well, friends, I am done asking myself this question, and you should be, too.

We're not alone in wanting to cut back on our alcohol. In a 2022 study, half of all drinkers said they planned to drink less, whether as a part of Dry January or just as a personal goal. But drinking less doesn't mean we want to feel like we're missing out on the camaraderie and socializing that so often comes with friends grabbing a few drinks. Mocktails are suddenly so hip because they offer a healthier, more inclusive, and more creative alternative to traditional cocktails. They are perfect for those of us who want to enjoy the flavors and ritual of a cocktail without the consequences or simply want to make healthier choices. Mocktails are having their moment, and it's time we ride the wave. And no, I'm not just saying that because I am a Florida gal.

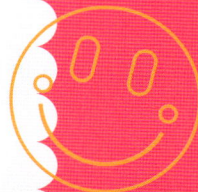

I grew tired of going to social events and feeling embarrassed by ordering "boring" drinks to sip on. This was when I recalled my own mantra, BYOE—Bring Your Own Energy. What was I thinking? Mocktails aren't boring; I just wasn't making them fun. So I jumped in the kitchen and started experimenting. Now known as the "mocktail queen" to my friends, family, and online community, I can think of no better way to celebrate my day than mixing up a quick sip. We don't ever have to settle for lackluster drinks. We're leaving boring behind and creating our own happy hour any day and any time.

I've brought all that fun to you in this book. *Mocktail Hour* makes it easy for you to celebrate every mood and every occasion. Just had a long day at work and you're in your comfiest pajamas about to watch your favorite show? Shake up a Coconut Cooler (page 85) or Nature's Lemonade (page 91) from my R&R recipes, starting on page 81. Picture yourself about to take a dip in the pool during those hot summer months as sweat drips down your back. Now picture a Lavender Haze Punch (page 128) in your hand. With *Mocktail Hour*, you'll discover that zero alcohol does not equal zero fun. By following these simple recipes and having a blast along the way, you can experience life's precious moments one sip at a time, without the headache.

Cheers to feeling good and making every hour a mocktail hour worth celebrating!

xo, Callie

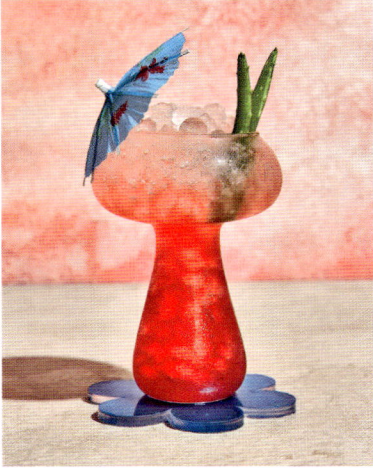
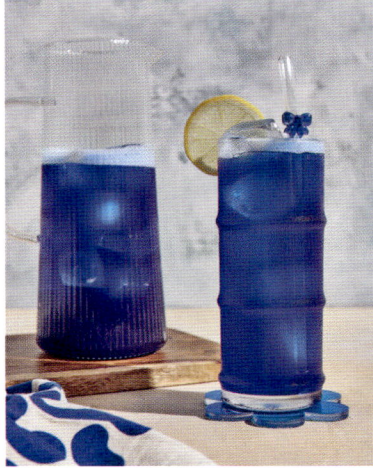
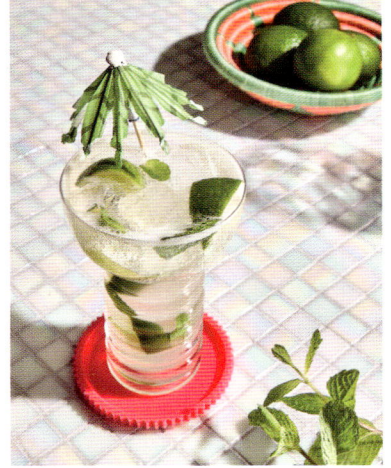
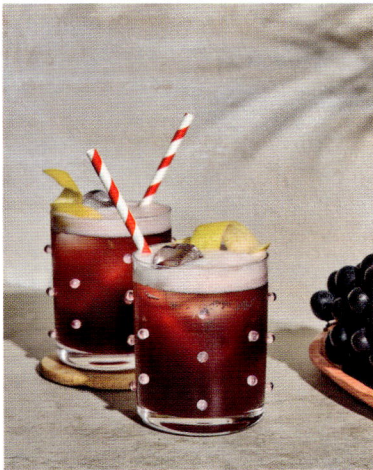
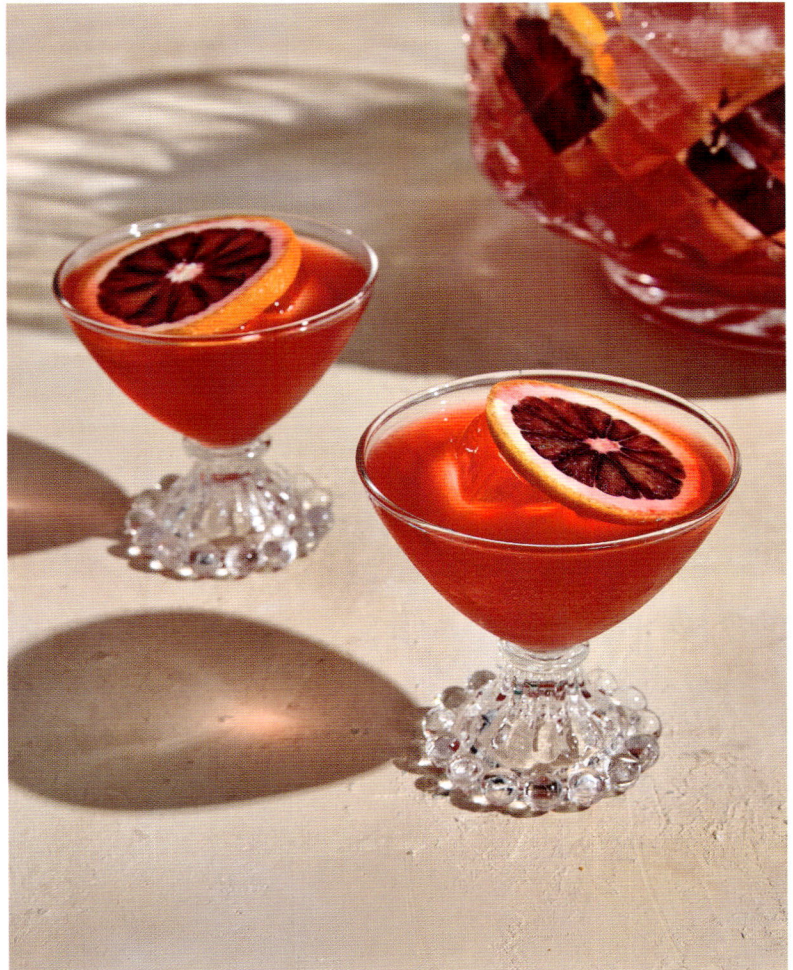
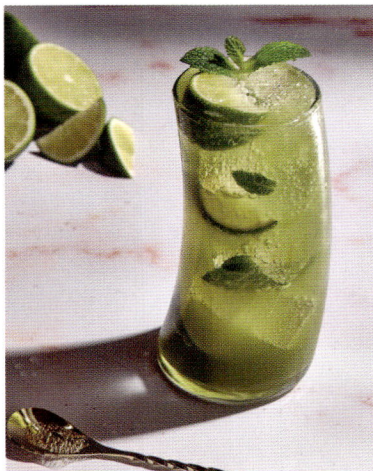

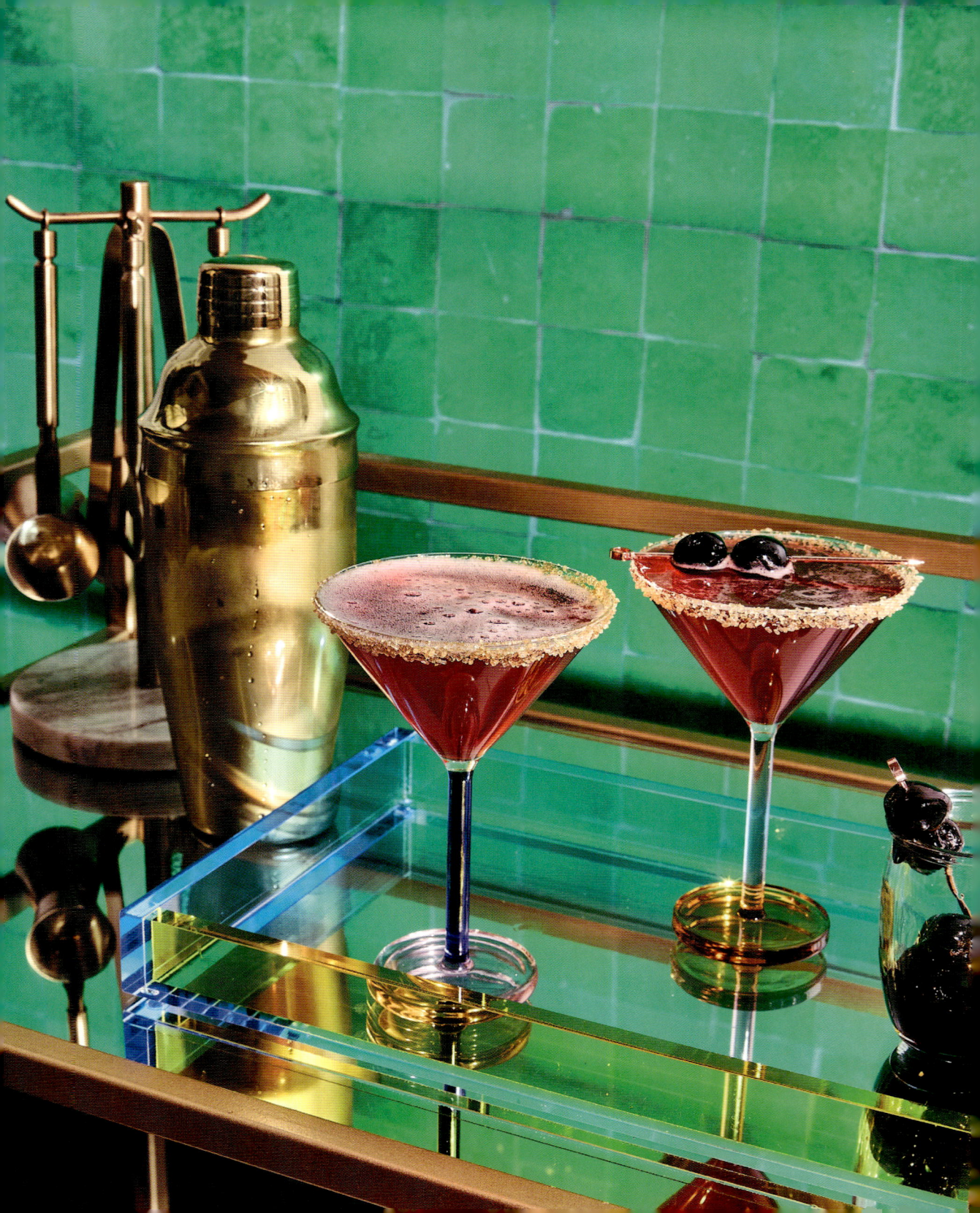

HOW TO USE THIS BOOK

If you've ever come across a fancy mocktail recipe and thought, *I don't have half of these ingredients*, don't worry: You're in the right place. This book is all about feeling confident in the kitchen (or wherever you're mixing up these yummy drinks). The goal is to make delicious, fun, and no-pressure mocktails with what you already have and feel good doing it.

Mocktail-making is best when you add your own twist and don't take it too seriously, which is how I live my life. So, let's talk about how to use this book in a way that works for you.

Make It Yours: Swaps and Substitutions

The perfect mocktail, at least for me, consists of about three ingredients: a juice or fruit, bubbles of some sort, and if you want to get fancy, some herbs, spices, and/or sweeteners. Mocktail-making is truly a DIY experience and I encourage you to get creative and mix up what sounds delicious and satisfying to you. Every recipe in this book is just a starting point. Don't have an ingredient? Swap it. Want it sweeter? Adjust it. Love a little spice? Throw it in.

Here are some quick swaps to keep in mind:

Sweeteners: Agave is my sweetener of choice in most of these recipes, but you can also use honey, maple syrup, or even a splash of juice to sweeten your drinks.

Bubbles: Club soda, sparkling water, ginger beer, sparkling coconut water, and kombucha are all great options.

Citrus: When a recipe calls for citrus, feel free to mix and match lemons, limes, oranges, and grapefruit.

Herbs: Basil, mint, and rosemary are three of my favorite herbs; fresh or dried, they all bring something special to your drink.

Spices: Turmeric, black pepper, ginger, and cinnamon add all the depth and complexity your tastebuds may be looking for.

There's no right or wrong way to do this, just *your* way.

Level It Up: Fun Additions and Tricks

Mocktails are more than just a drink; they're an experience. One of my favorite parts of mocktail-making is getting creative with the presentation. Make them extra special with these easy tricks.

Ice cubes: Freeze juices, herbs, or edible flowers into your ice for a surprise burst of flavor. And don't even get me started on all the fun ice molds you can use to shape them.

Rim it up: For the rim of your glass, use sugar, salt, Tajín, or crushed freeze-dried fruit. You can even add citrus zest into your salt. Do whatever makes you happy!

Frozen fruit: Skip ice altogether and use frozen fruits in your drinks instead. I love using berries, cherries, pineapple, mango, and grapes! Use any extra fruit to make smoothies!

Garnishes: There are so many amazing garnish options: fresh herbs, citrus twists, candy canes, a skewer of gummy bears, and more. How fun, right?

Zero-proof or alcohol-removed spirits: Since I wanted these recipes to be easily made with ingredients we all have in our kitchens, I purposely left out zero-proof spirits (with the exception of the Bellini Me, Please on page 139). However, feel free to add these ingredients to any recipe you see fit.

Confidence in Mocktail-Making

This book isn't just about mixing drinks; it's about mixing confidence into everything you do. The most important thing is that you're having fun doing it.

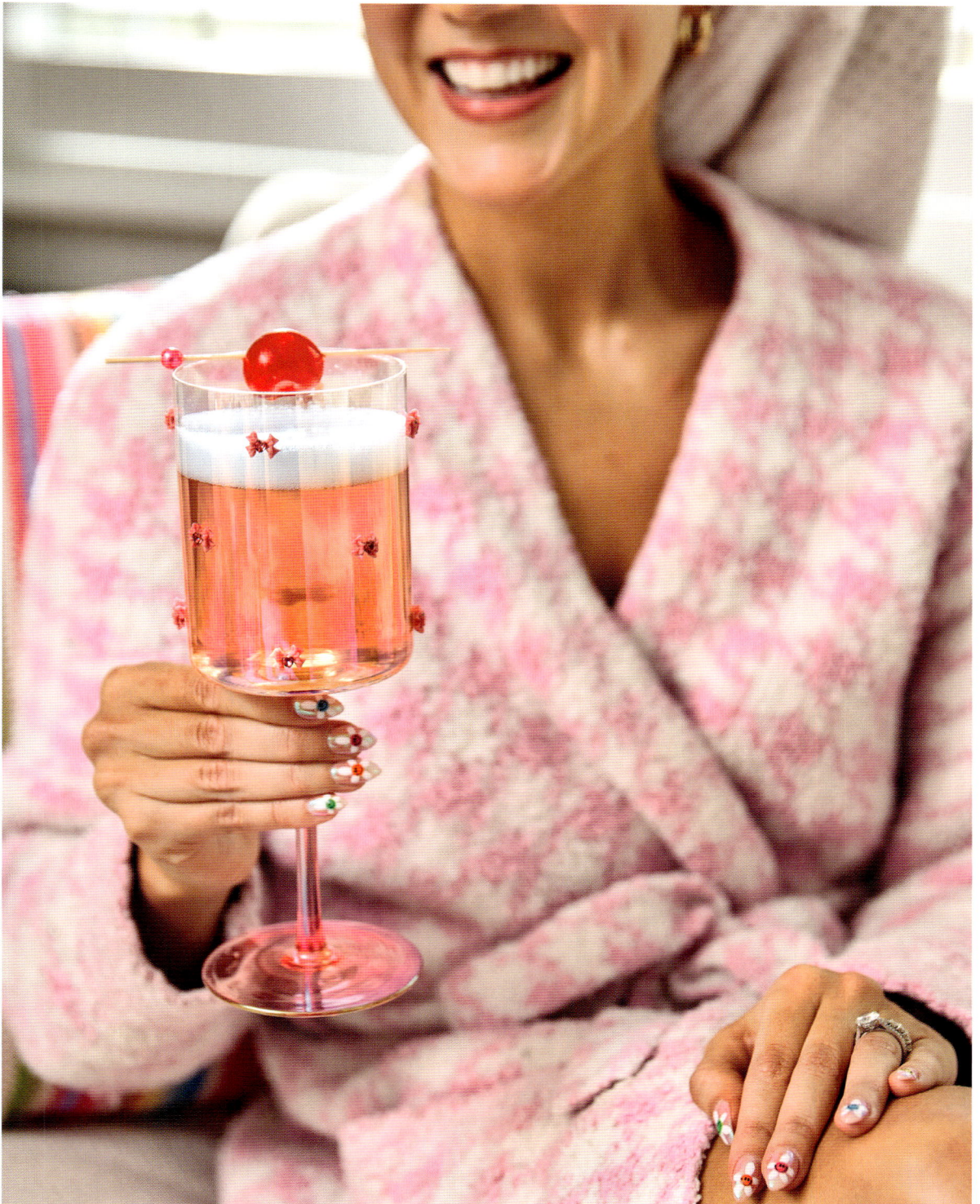

- Don't worry about making your drink perfect; worry about making it yours.

- Use what's in your fridge; if you don't have a specific ingredient, that's okay!

- Sip, experiment, and trust yourself.

- Remember, we all have different taste buds, so if someone doesn't like a drink you make, you can just drink theirs (hehe)!

By the time you finish this book, you'll be whipping up mocktails with confidence and truly feeling *good*. Now grab your favorite glass, pick a recipe, and let's get to living our best life!

GETTING STARTED

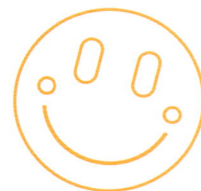

Setting Up Your Bar Cart

Just like a well-stocked kitchen makes choosing what to eat a lot easier (or harder, if you're indecisive like I am), a well-stocked bar cart makes mocktail-making effortless and fun. Think of it as part of your self-care toolkit, ready to help you unwind, celebrate, or just make hydration a little more exciting.

You'll only need a few tools to sip your way into confidence and feeling good. Here's what you'll want to have on hand.

Shaker & stirrer: Blend flavors seamlessly, whether you're going for smooth or fizzy.

Citrus juicer: Fresh lemon or lime juice makes all the difference. Squeezing by hand just isn't as fun.

Measuring tools: Use a jigger or small measuring cups, because balance is key in drinks and in life.

Strainer: Keep things clean and crisp by straining out pulp and seeds.

Blender: A necessary tool for blended mocktails, blenders are great to keep in the kitchen.

Glasses: Use what makes you feel good: fancy coupe glasses, a mason jar, or even your favorite everyday cup.

Garnish station: Fresh herbs and citrus slices go a long way.

With just these few essentials, you'll be ready to stir, shake, and sip your way to delicious, confidence-boosting mocktails, because feeling good should always taste good, too!

Get to Know Your Glassware

Just like a bright outfit sets the mood for an occasion, the right glass can elevate your mocktail experience. But don't overthink it. There are no rules here! This is not a regular mocktail book; it's a cool mocktail book.

The glass you choose can change the vibe of your drink, from cozy and casual to sleek and sophisticated. Here's a quick guide to finding your match.

Coupe glass: Elegant and timeless, perfect for bubbly or shaken drinks that deserve a little flair. I use these every opportunity I can.

Highball glass: Tall and refreshing, ideal for drinks with lots of fizz and fun garnishes.

Lowball/rocks glass: Short and sturdy, great for bold and flavorful sips over ice.

Mug: For warm mocktails or just because it's your favorite comfort cup.

Wineglass: Fancy but versatile; perfect for spritzes, fruit-infused mocktails, or just feeling extra.

Martini glass: Sleek, chic, and classic. Designed for ice-free drinks, to keep your mocktail crisp while making you feel fancy.

At the end of the day, you do you when it comes to whatever glass you want to use!

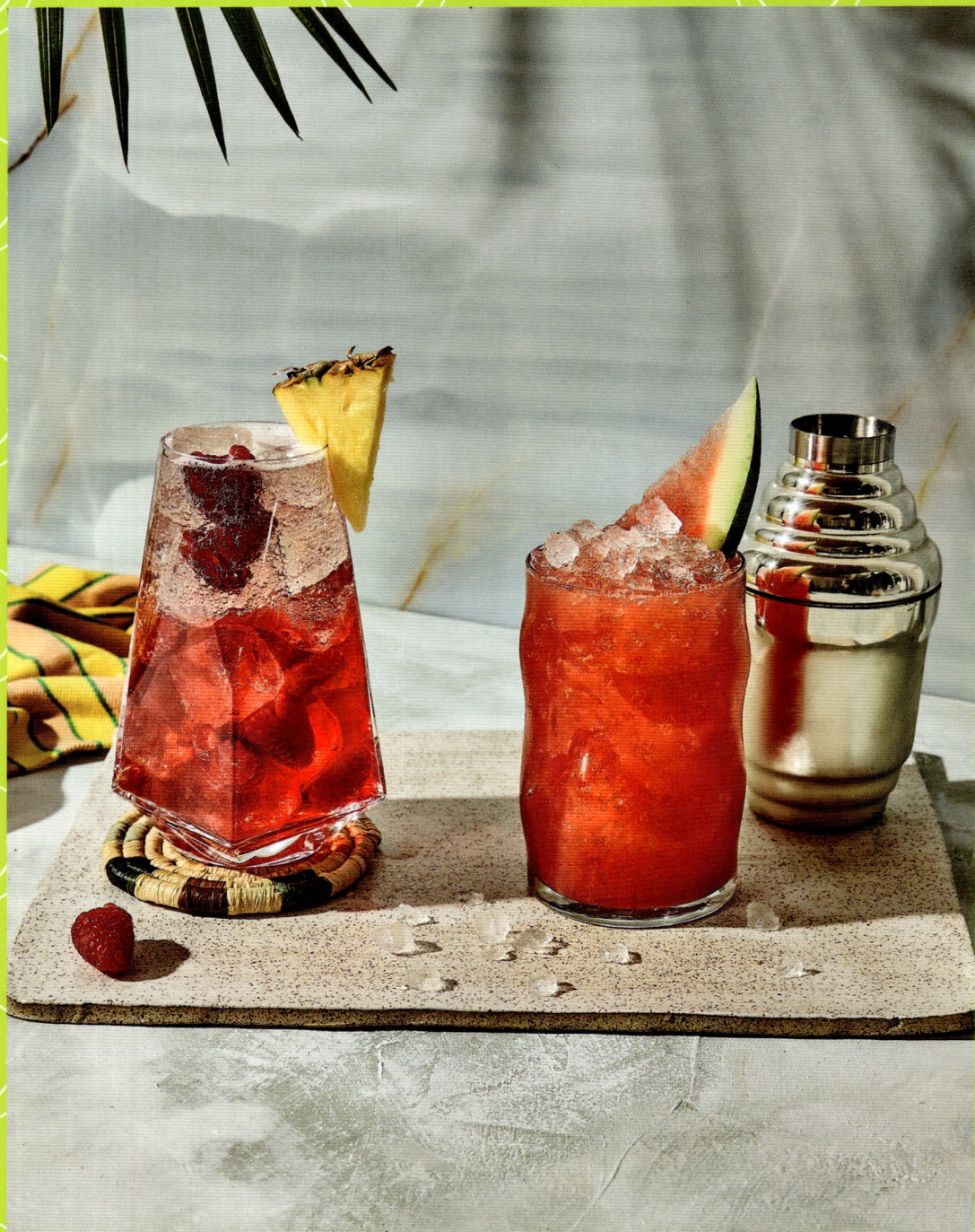

CHAPTER ONE

ENERGY
Elixirs

I truly believe energy is everything, and these mocktails are packed with just that. Turn to this chapter whenever you need a boost and a reminder to bring your own energy. BYOE, baby!

EYE PATCHES
& Espresso

SERVES 1

Ice cubes

½ cup tonic water

1 shot espresso

1 orange slice, for garnish

1. Fill a lowball glass with ice.

2. Pour the tonic water into the glass and top with the espresso shot. Garnish with an orange slice.

WANT IT SWEETER? Add agave syrup to taste.

To make an **ORANGE ESPRESSO TONIC**, add orange juice to taste.

To make a **SHIRLEY TEMPLE ESPRESSO TONIC**, add grenadine to taste.

Some people start their day with coffee. I start mine with coffee and under-eye patches, because self-care is a full-time job. Eye Patches & Espresso is a go-to for when I'm looking to wake up and spruce things up. A drink as energizing as it is sophisticated, it makes you feel like you have your life together, even if you're still rocking your eye patches.

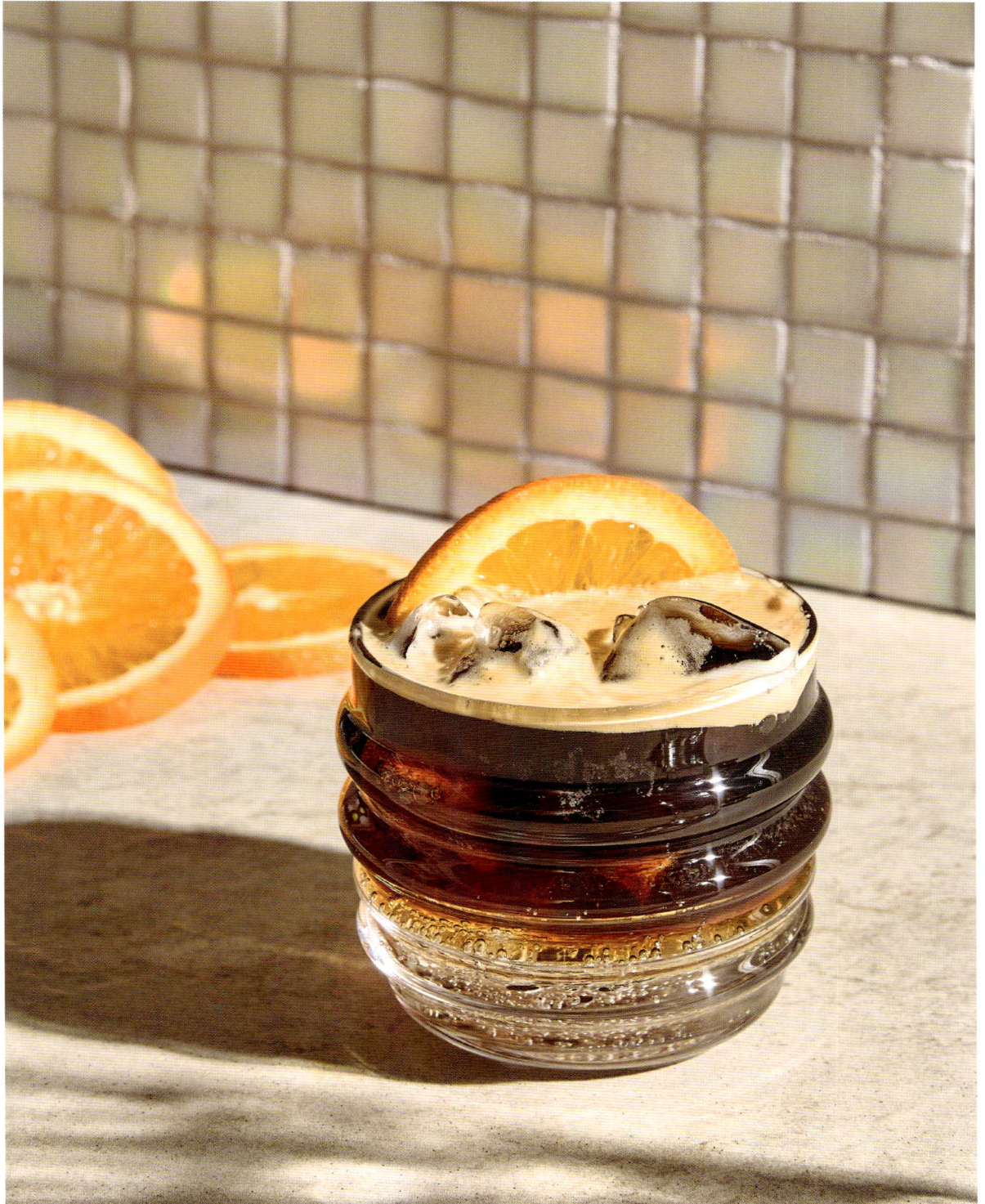

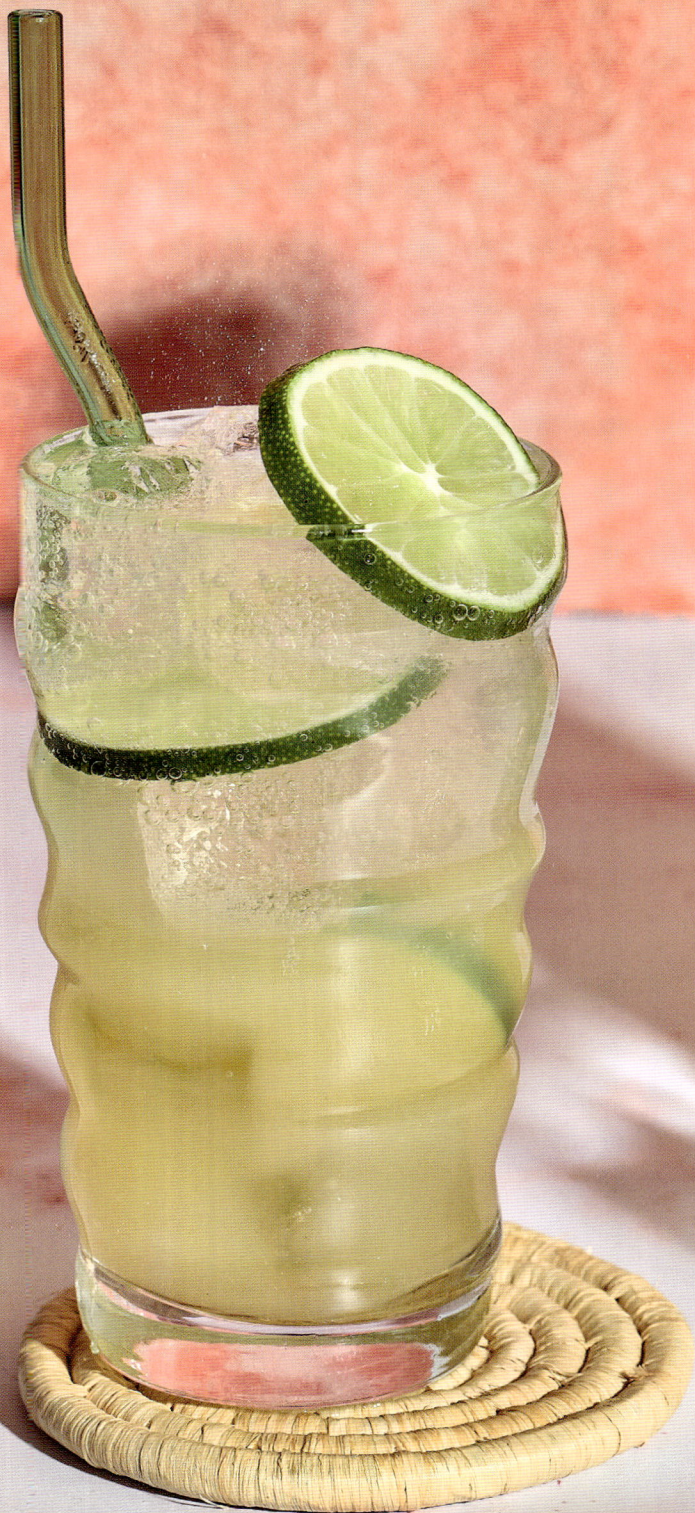

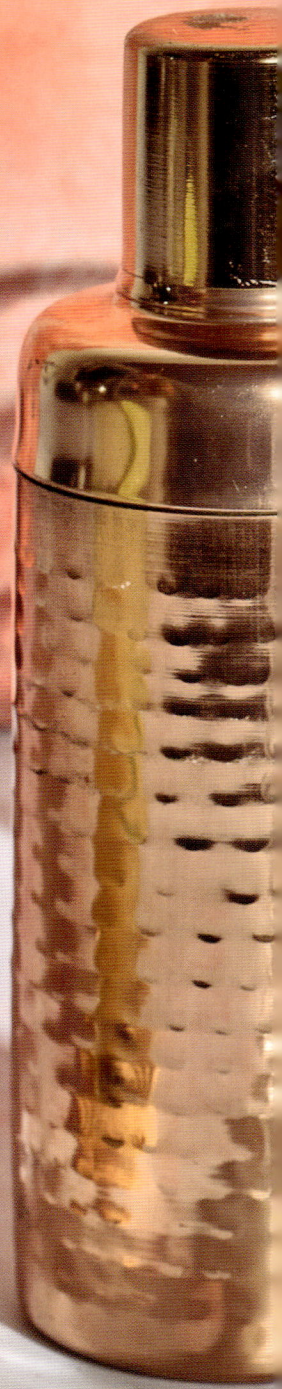

GINGER LIMEADE

BEND & (Ginger) Snap

SERVES 1

Juice of 1½ limes

¼ cup water

1½ teaspoons freshly grated ginger

Ice cubes

1 cup lime sparkling water

Lime slices, for garnish

1. Pour the lime juice and water into a shaker. Add the ginger and a handful of ice.

2. Shake until the outside of the shaker is frosty, about 5 seconds.

3. Fill a highball glass with ice. (I prefer to fill it to the brim.)

4. Strain the mixture into the glass. If you prefer to remove the ginger pulp, strain through a mesh strainer.

5. Top with the sparkling water, then garnish with the lime slices.

This is not your typical limeade but, wow, it's delicious. The ginger packs quite the punch and is great for digestion. I had the idea for this drink after an experience my husband Chris and I had in Bali when I was 7 weeks pregnant. One night, I was feeling nauseous, so I tried to cancel our dinner reservation by telling the restaurant that Chris was sick (I didn't tell him this). Long story short, we ended up not canceling. At the restaurant, the waitress kept asking Chris if he was feeling okay, leaving him very confused. At the end of the meal, the manager offered Chris some ginger tea and said it would make his stomach feel better. That's when I admitted that I had tried to blame him for canceling our reservation. Whoops!

GRAPEFRUIT PALOMA

Positive Vibes
PALOMA

SERVES 1

½ cup grapefruit juice

Juice of ½ lime

1 teaspoon agave syrup, to taste (optional)

Ice cubes

½ cup club soda

GARNISH

Coarse salt

2 lime wedges

1 grapefruit slice

1. Pour a thin layer of salt onto a small plate. Rub a lime wedge around the rim of a rocks glass, then dip the rim into the salt by rotating and rolling.

2. Pour the grapefruit juice, lime juice, and agave syrup (if using) into the glass. Stir, then add your preferred amount of ice.

3. Top with club soda, then garnish with a grapefruit slice and a lime wedge.

Calling all paloma lovers: This mocktail is for you! I'm going to be honest: I've had maybe one or two tequila-based palomas in my life, but grapefruit juice has my heart, so I knew I needed to make a mocktail version. If you like some spice, add some sliced jalapeños into your glass and muddle before topping with club soda. If you love grapefruit like I do, try the So Fetch Spritz (page 68) or Spice Up Your Life (page 57).

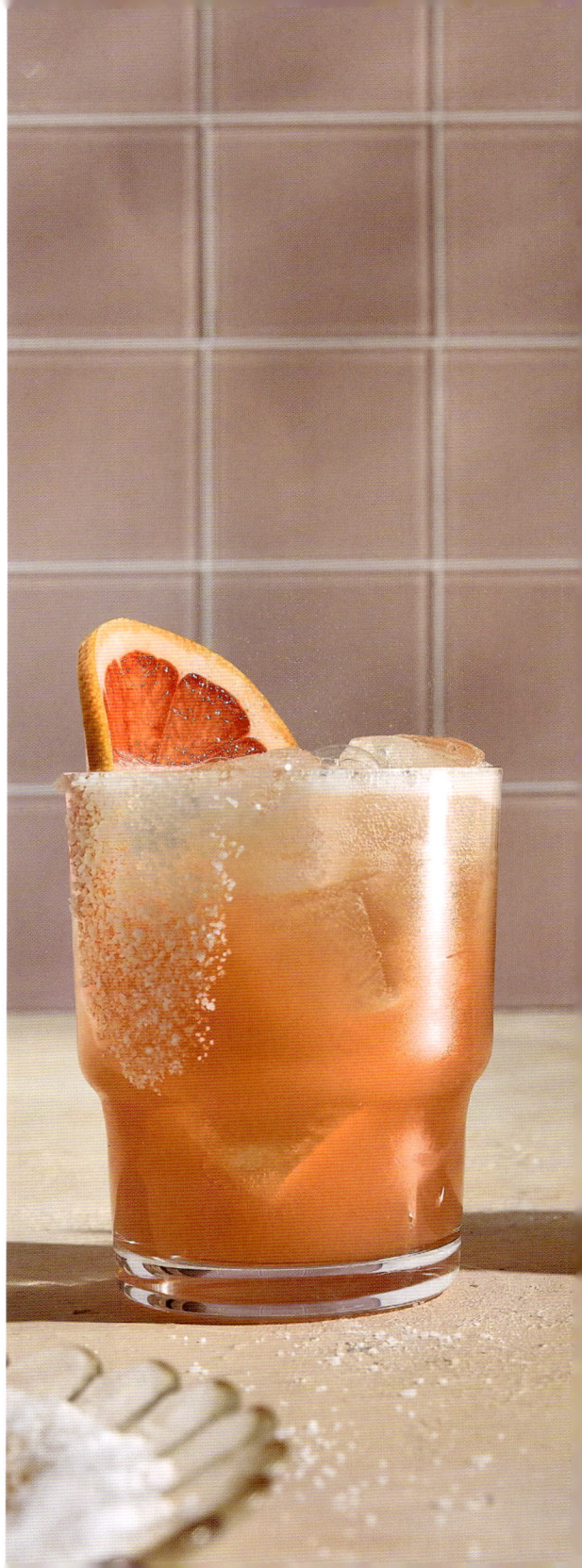

CARROT ORANGE REFRESHER

SUNNY
Roots

SERVES 1

½ cup carrot juice

½ cup orange juice

Juice of ½ lemon

1 tablespoon agave syrup

Ice cubes

¼ cup unflavored sparkling water

GARNISH

1 mint sprig

1 carrot ribbon

1. Combine the carrot juice, orange juice, lemon juice, agave syrup, and a handful of ice in a shaker.

2. Shake until the outside of the shaker is frosty, about 5 seconds.

3. Add a handful of ice to a rocks glass. Pour the juice mixture over the ice.

4. Top with sparkling water and stir well.

5. Garnish with a mint sprig and a carrot ribbon.

Let me introduce you to your new favorite way to make your orange juice that much sunnier. This vibrant drink supports glowing skin, a happy immune system, and all-around good vibes, which we know is the root of feeling your best. Because when you shine on the inside, it shows on the outside.

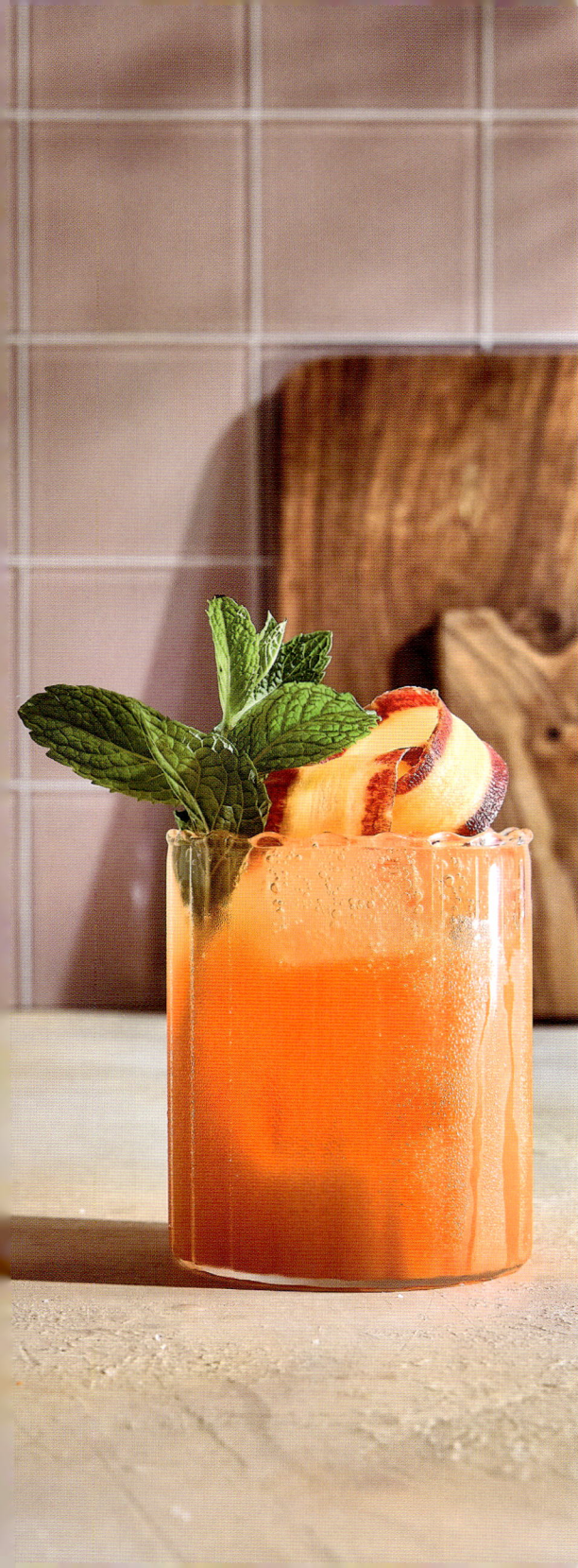

ZEN GREEN *Mojito*

SERVES 1

1 teaspoon ceremonial-grade matcha powder (see Tip)

¼ cup hot water (about 175°F)

1 tablespoon agave syrup

1 lime, cut into wedges

10 to 12 mint leaves

Ice cubes

½ cup unflavored sparkling water

GARNISH

1 mint sprig

1 lime wedge

1. Combine the matcha powder and hot water in a small bowl.

2. Whisk the matcha in a Z motion until it is frothy or bubbles. Whisk in the agave, then set aside.

3. Place the mint leaves and lime wedges in a tall glass and muddle, using a muddler or the back of a wooden spoon, by pressing gently and twisting 3 to 5 times, just enough to release the mint flavor without tearing the leaves.

4. Fill the glass with ice, then pour in the matcha mixture.

5. Top with sparkling water and stir gently.

6. Garnish with a mint sprig and a lime wedge to make it more fun!

TIP If you have a strainer, you can sift the matcha powder to remove clumps.

Listen, if there is one drink I'm making many variations of, it's going to be a mojito. Mint with a side of energy—SAY LESS. If you like this, you'll love the Basilina Buzz (page 157).

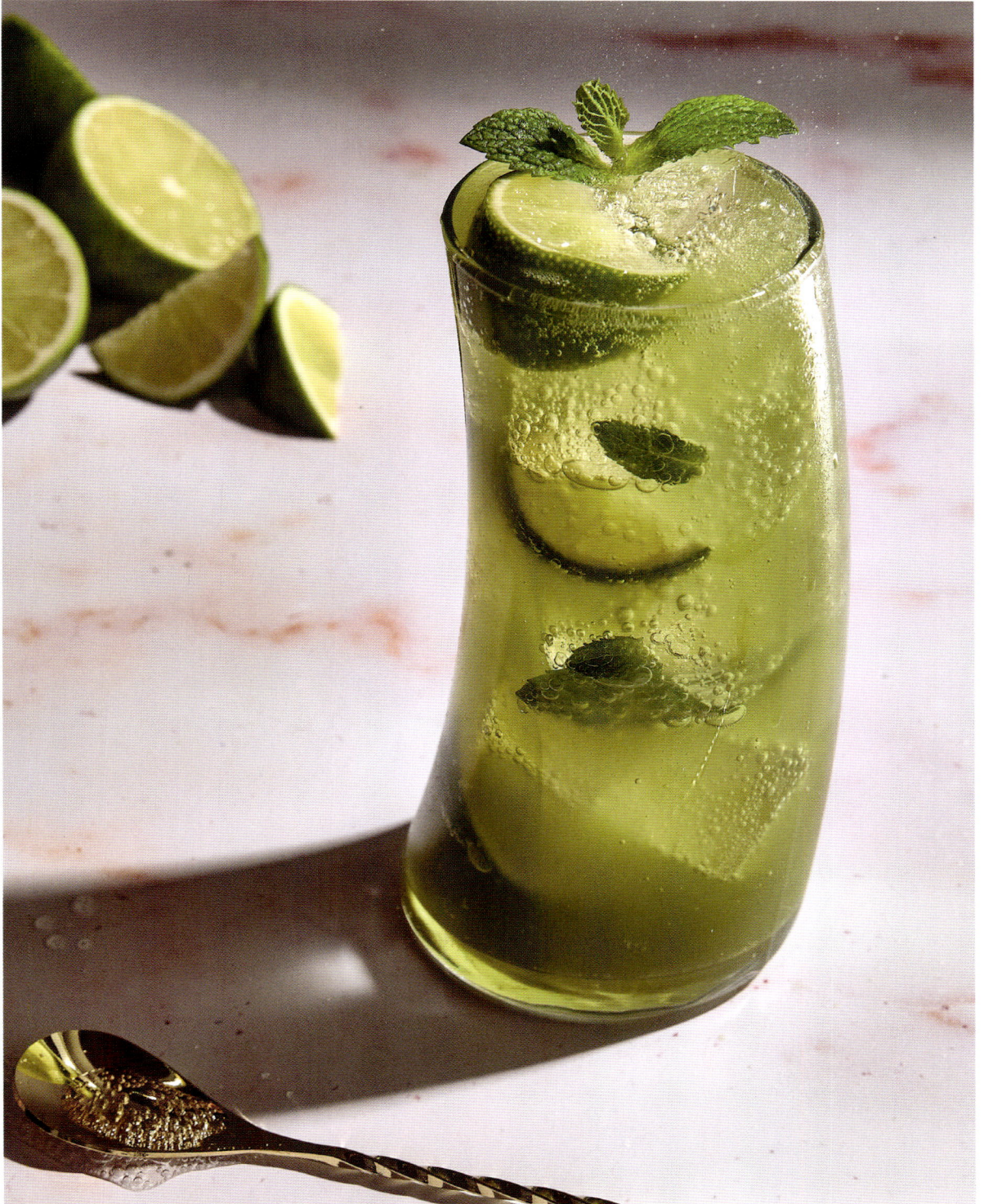

IT'S GIVING
Fresh

SERVES 1

1 cup cubed watermelon (see Note)

½ cup water

½ cup brewed green tea, chilled

Juice of ½ lime

2 teaspoons agave syrup (optional)

Ice cubes

1 watermelon wedge, for garnish

1. Blend the watermelon and water in a blender until smooth.

2. Use a mesh strainer to strain the watermelon puree into a shaker. Discard the pulp.

3. Add the green tea, lime juice, agave (if using), and a handful of ice. Shake until the outside is frosty, about 10 seconds.

4. Fill a tall glass with ice cubes, then strain the watermelon mixture into the glass. Garnish with a watermelon wedge.

NOTE You can also use ½ cup store-bought watermelon juice instead of the cubed watermelon and water and skip to step 3.

Is there anything more refreshing than biting into a juicy watermelon chunk? NOPE. The hydrating watermelon and crisp green tea in this drink is truly a match made in heaven. If you like watermelon, you'll also love the Watermelon Sugar (page 46).

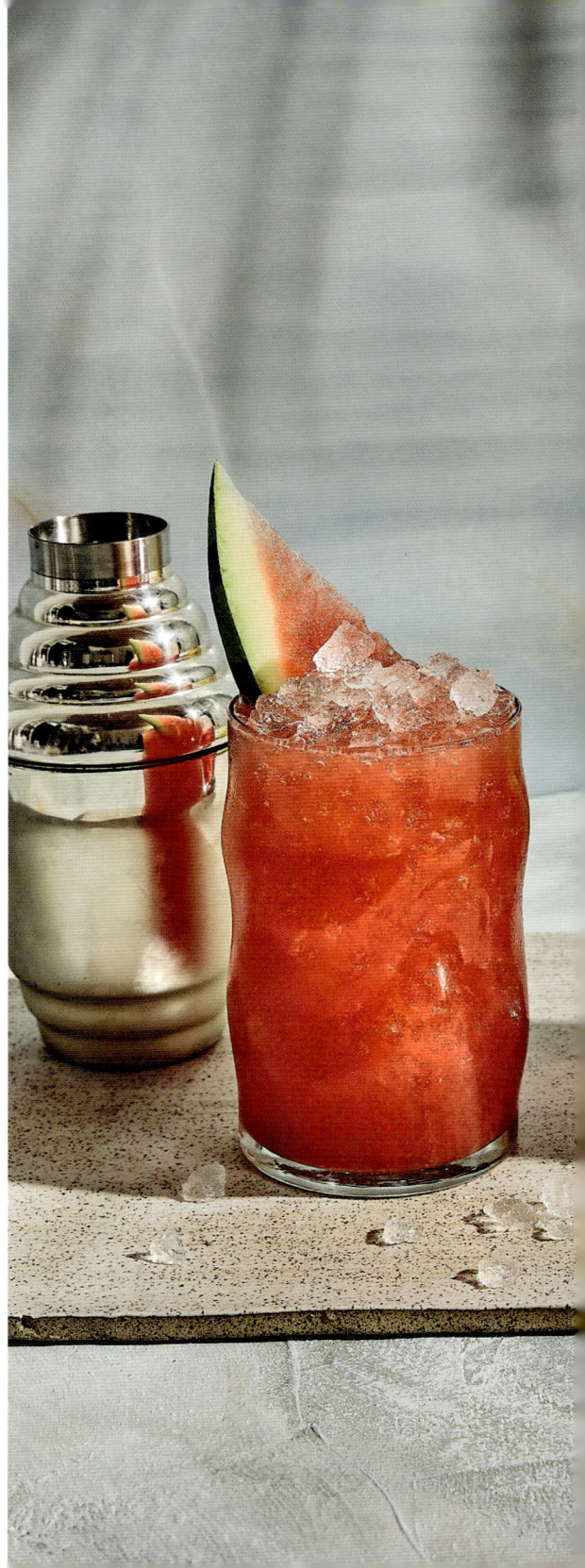

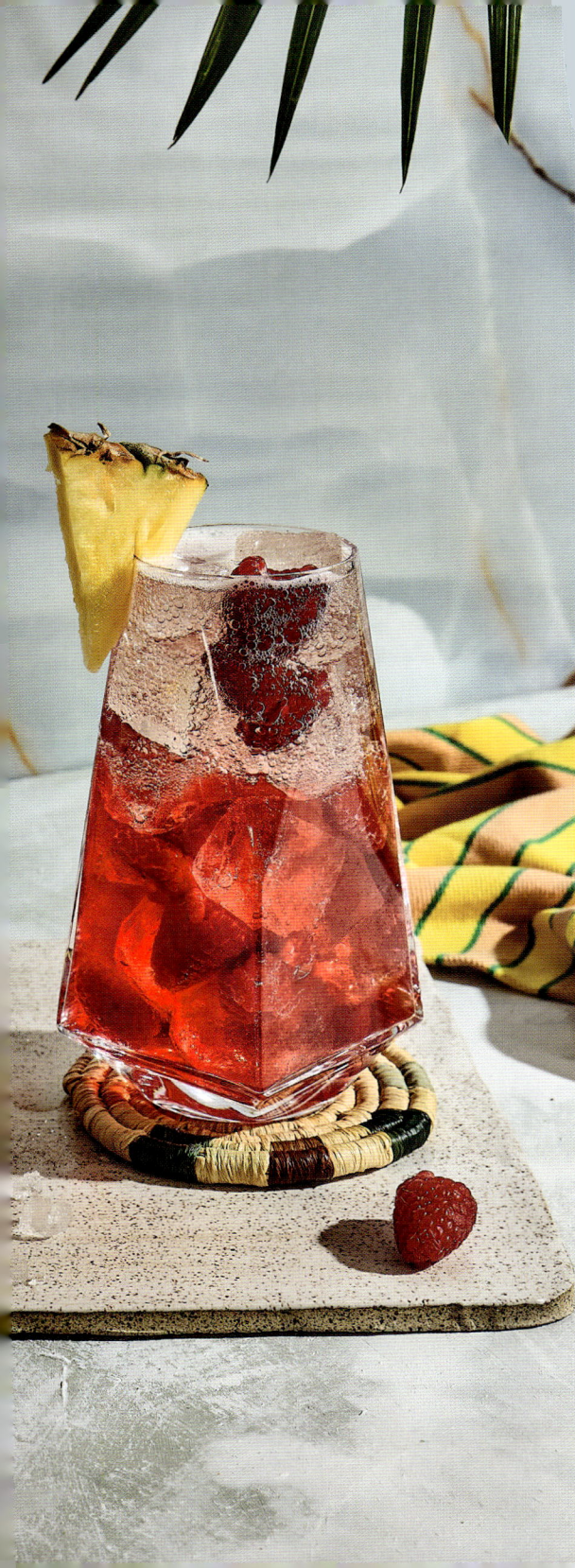

SPARKLING HIBISCUS BERRY TEA

BLOOMING
Boost

SERVES 1

1 cup water	Ice cubes
2 hibiscus tea bags	¼ cup lemon sparkling water
2 tablespoons honey	
Handful of raspberries	1 pineapple slice, for garnish

1. Bring the water to a boil in a kettle.

2. Pour into a cup, add the tea bags, and steep for 5 to 7 minutes.

3. Add the honey, stir, and set aside to cool to room temperature.

4. Place the raspberries in a tall glass and muddle, using a muddler or the back of a wooden spoon, pressing gently and twisting until the berries break apart and the juices release.

5. Add ice cubes to the brim, then add the tea and stir well.

6. Top with sparkling water, then garnish with a pineapple slice for a pop of energy.

Next time you consider sending someone flowers, remember you have this recipe and can send this to them instead. This drink is tart and juicy, packed with antioxidants and a touch of natural energy. Sip on this and get ready to bloom into your best self.

Energy Elixers

29

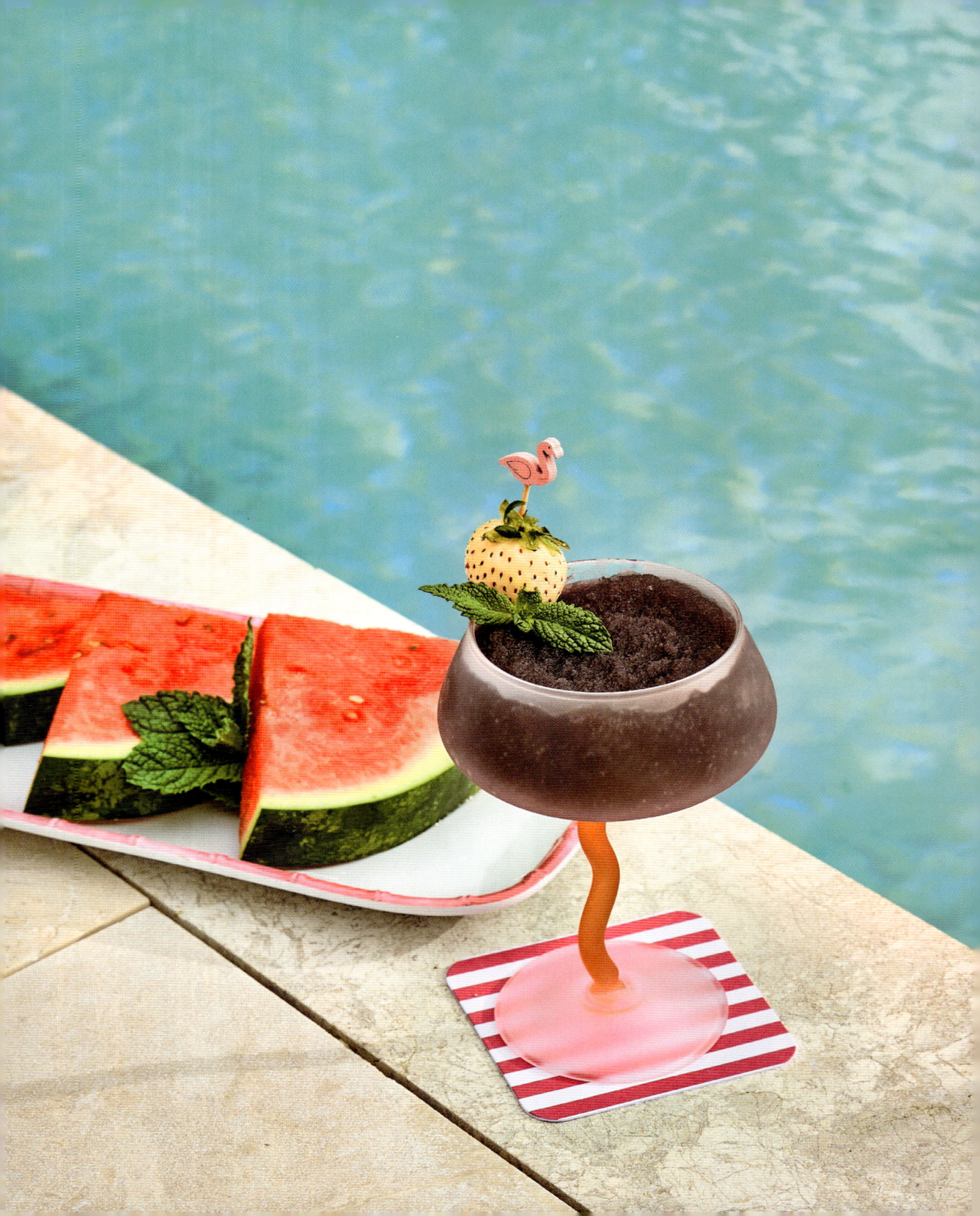

BERRY ME
in Acai

SERVES 1

One 3.5-ounce packet frozen acai puree (see Tip)

4 frozen strawberries

¼ cup coconut water

1 pitted date (optional)

3 or 4 ice cubes

Mint sprigs, for garnish

1. Combine the acai puree, strawberries, coconut water, date (if using), and ice in a blender. Blend until smooth.

2. Pour the mixture into a coupe glass and garnish with mint sprigs.

TIP To thaw the acai packet before blending, run it under hot water for 20 seconds and then break it apart or leave it at room temperature for 5 to 10 minutes.

Did anyone else go through a phase where they had an acai bowl every day, or was it just me? I was obsessed, and if my wallet allowed me, I still would be. Sweet, tangy, and packed with antioxidants, this is the daiquiri you didn't know you needed. The strawberries keep it tart while the date keeps it sweet, so feel free to adjust to your liking. I also like to swap in blueberries for the strawberries—give that a try if you have frozen blueberries on hand!

SPILL THE TEA
Tini

SERVES 1

1 cup water

1 jasmine tea bag (see Note)

Juice of 1 lemon

1 tablespoon honey

Handful of ice cubes

¼ cup tonic water

Lemon twist, for garnish

1. Bring the water to a boil in a kettle.

2. Pour into a cup, then add the tea bag and steep for 2 to 4 minutes. Set aside to cool to room temperature.

3. Combine the tea, lemon juice, honey, and ice in a shaker. Shake until the outside of the shaker is frosty, about 5 seconds.

4. Strain the mixture into a martini glass.

5. Top with tonic water, then garnish with a lemon twist.

NOTE For a stronger, more bitter flavor, add another tea bag.

Everyone loves tea and martinis, so why not enjoy them together in one glass? The soothing jasmine tea and bold elegance of a martini create a sip just as uplifting as it is refreshing. So, grab your girls and spill the tea, but only the good stuff.

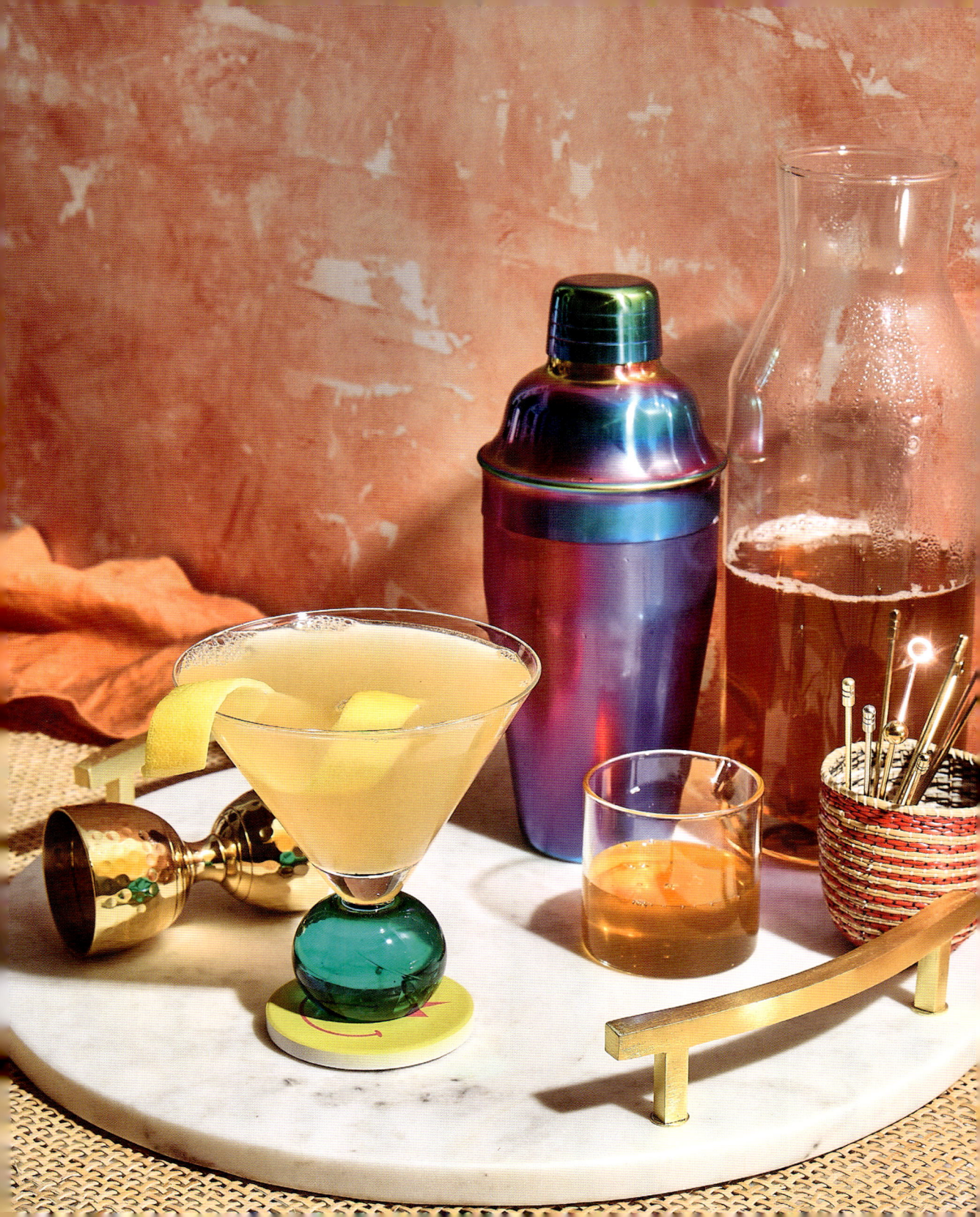

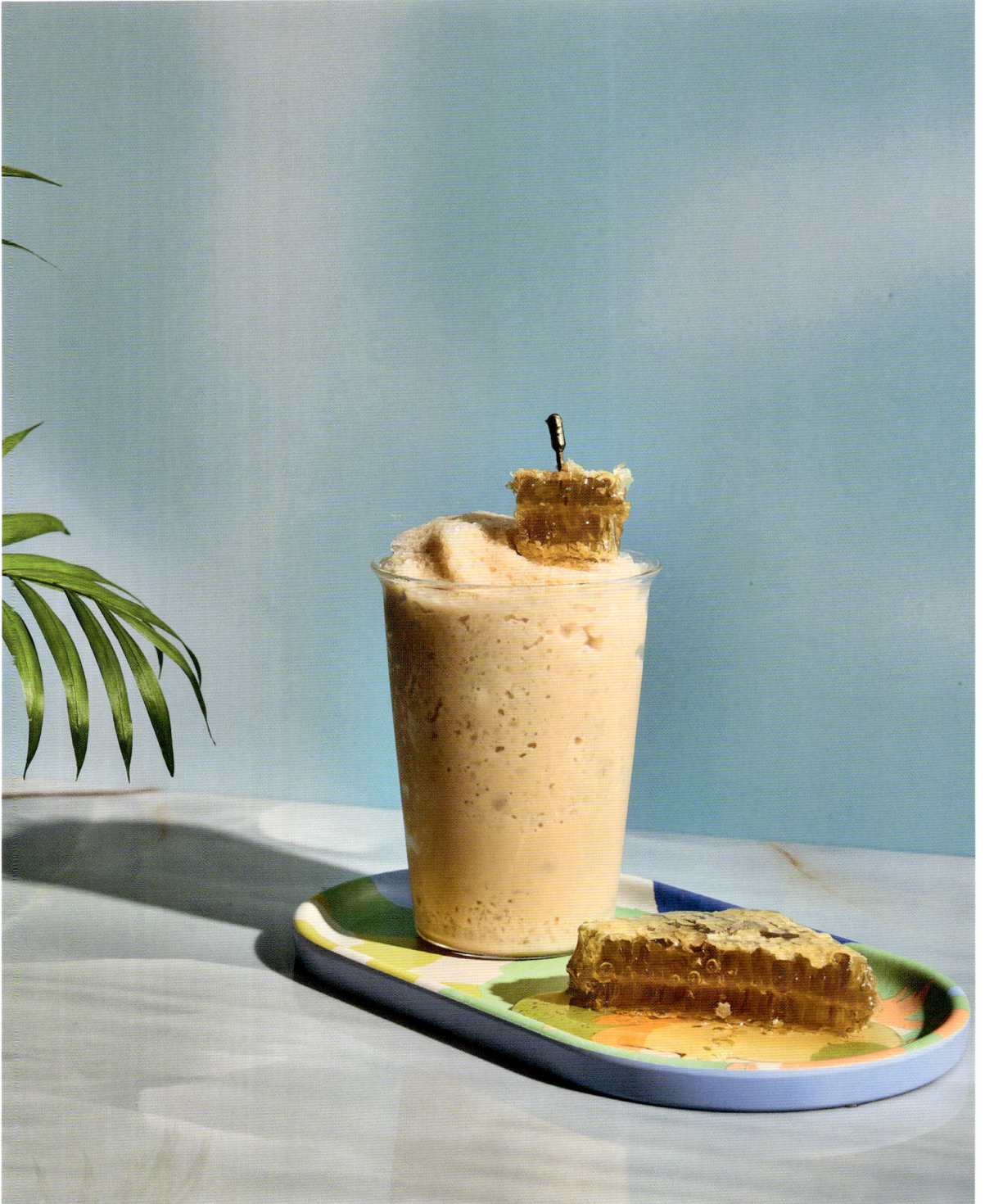

FRAP *Queen*

SERVES 1

1 cup brewed chai tea, cooled

½ cup milk of choice, frozen into ice cubes

1 tablespoon maple syrup, or to taste

½ teaspoon vanilla extract

GARNISH

Ground cinnamon

Honeycomb chunks (optional)

1. Combine the tea, milk ice cubes, maple syrup, and vanilla in a blender.

2. Blend until smooth, then pour into a highball glass.

3. Sprinkle cinnamon on top and add honeycomb (if using). Sip through a straw or use a spoon to enjoy.

Frap and yap gals unite! Bow down to the Frap Queen, where chai spices meet creamy goodness in a frappe fit for royalty. Don't tell my dog Charly; she thinks she's the only queen, and I'm not going to be the person to break it to her. For a bolder chai flavor, use chai concentrate in place of chai tea.

TEN QUICK
Energy-Boosting Ideas

Move like nobody's watching. Stand up and move your body.

Sip, Sip, Hooray for H2O. Invest in a water bottle you like and sip it up!

Snack queens unite. Make a superfood snack to replenish those energy levels and wake you up.

Embrace the power of naps. A power nap really does wonders for me.

Zen out. Take a moment to close your eyes and find your breath.

Chase the sunlight. Soak up all the sunshine or sit near a window to chase away the energy-zapping shadows.

Laugh. Put on a fun show, listen to a lighthearted podcast, or simply just laugh with a friend or significant other.

Caffeinate. Treat yourself to a coffee or matcha date with a friend or even have a solo lunch date for intention-setting and reflecting.

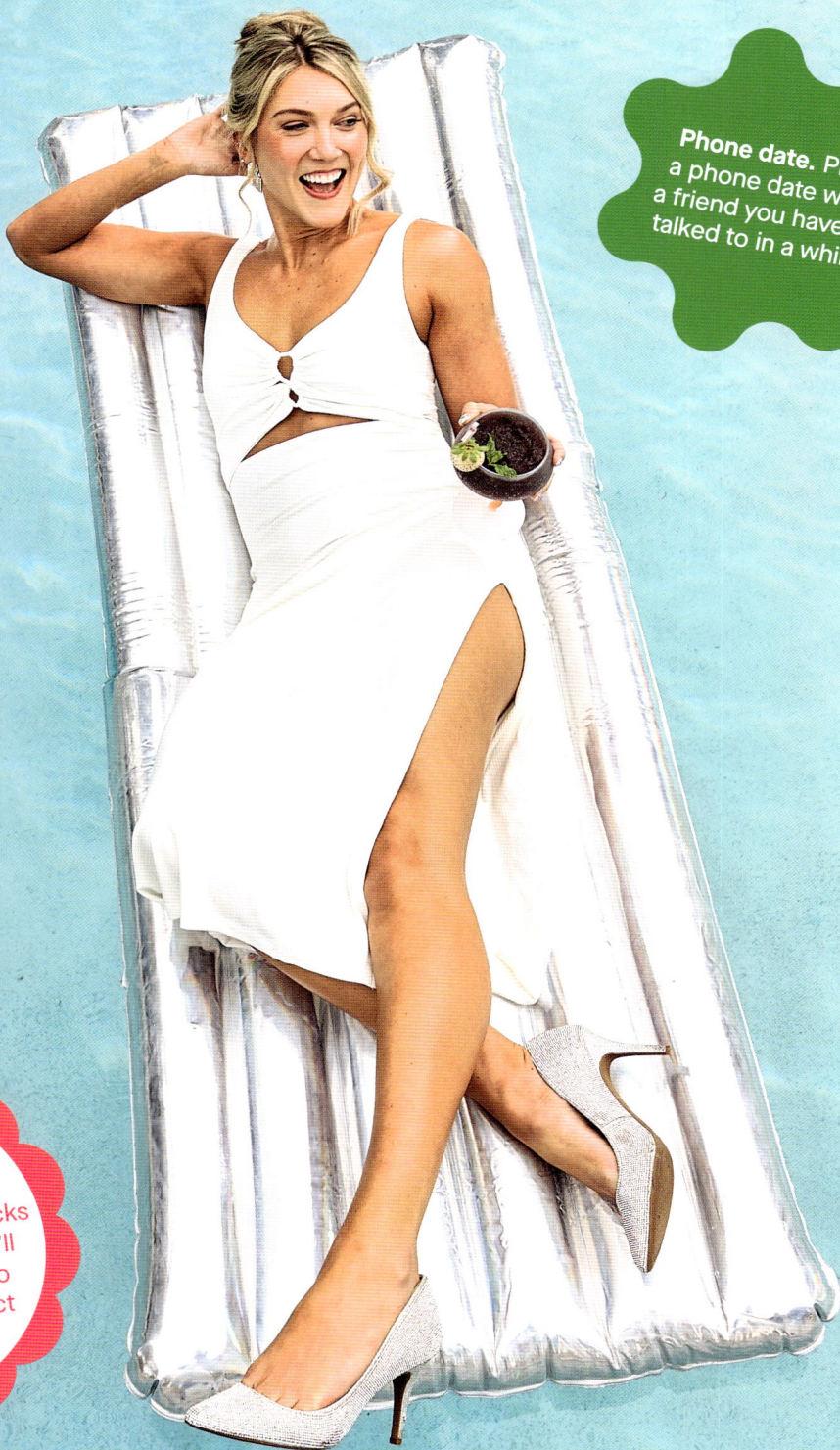

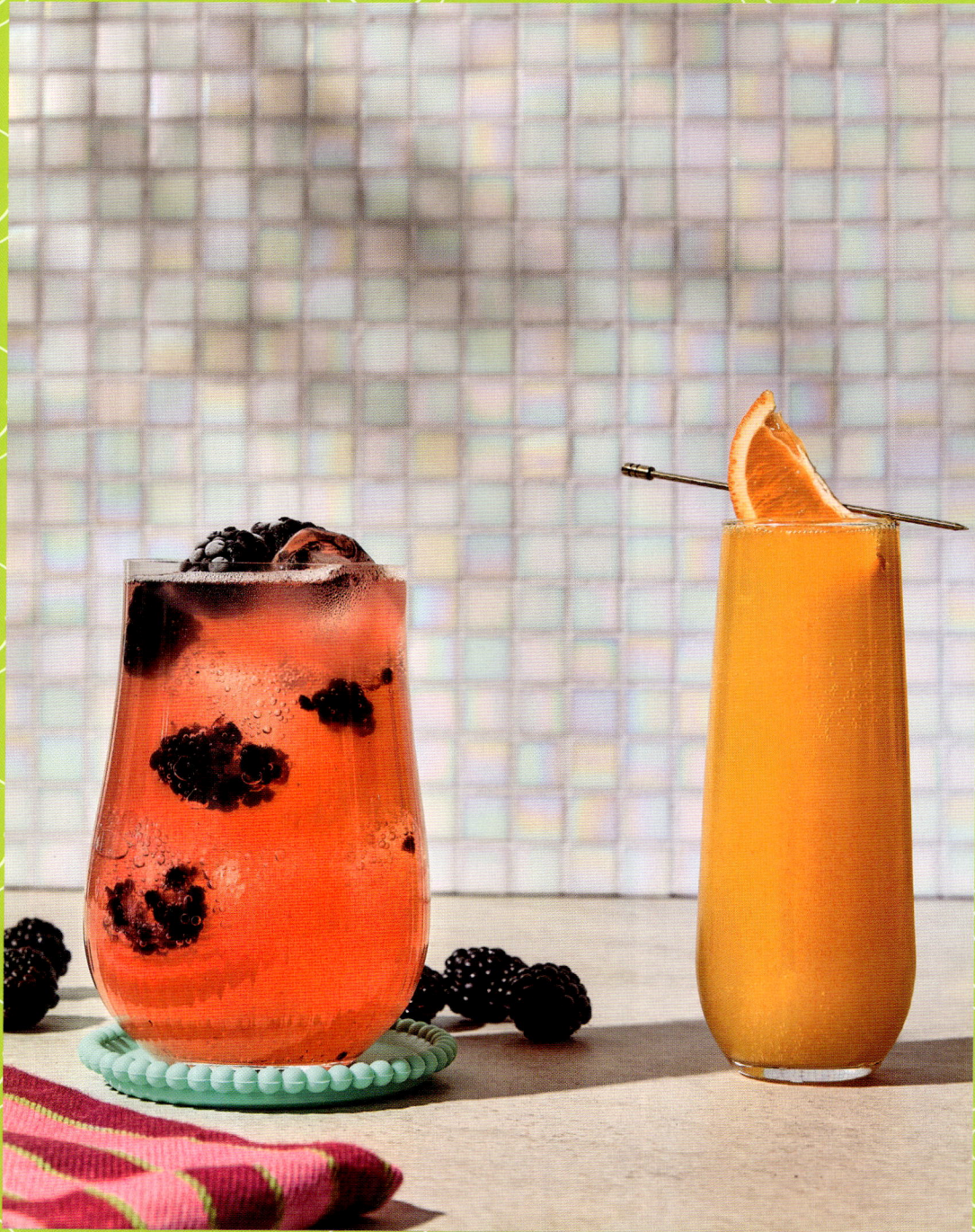

CHAPTER TWO

MOOD
Boosters

Sometimes life comes at you hard. These drinks won't solve all your problems, but they sure will help—just like listening to your favorite pop song.

THANK YOU, *Next,*

SERVES 1

¼ cup orange juice

Juice of 1 lime

2 teaspoons hot honey

1 jalapeño, sliced, divided

Ice cubes

1 cup club soda

GARNISH

2 lime wedges, divided

Tajín

1. Coat the rim of a coupe or rocks glass with a lime wedge. Pour the Tajín onto a small plate, then dip the rim into it to coat.

2. Combine the orange juice, lime juice, hot honey, and half of the jalapeño in a shaker. Muddle, using a muddler or the back of a wooden spoon, until the jalapeño is broken down and aromatic, 5 to 10 twists.

3. Add a handful of ice cubes to the shaker and shake until the outside of the shaker is frosty, about 5 seconds.

4. Fill the glass with ice. Strain the margarita into the glass.

5. Top with club soda, then garnish with the remaining jalapeño and lime wedge.

This spicy marg mocktail is all about moving on, glowing up, and leaving bad energy behind—and we have Ariana to thank for that. With zesty lime, jalapeño heat, and a touch of sweetness, we will have no time for bad vibes—only good sips, good company, and a little spice to keep things interesting.

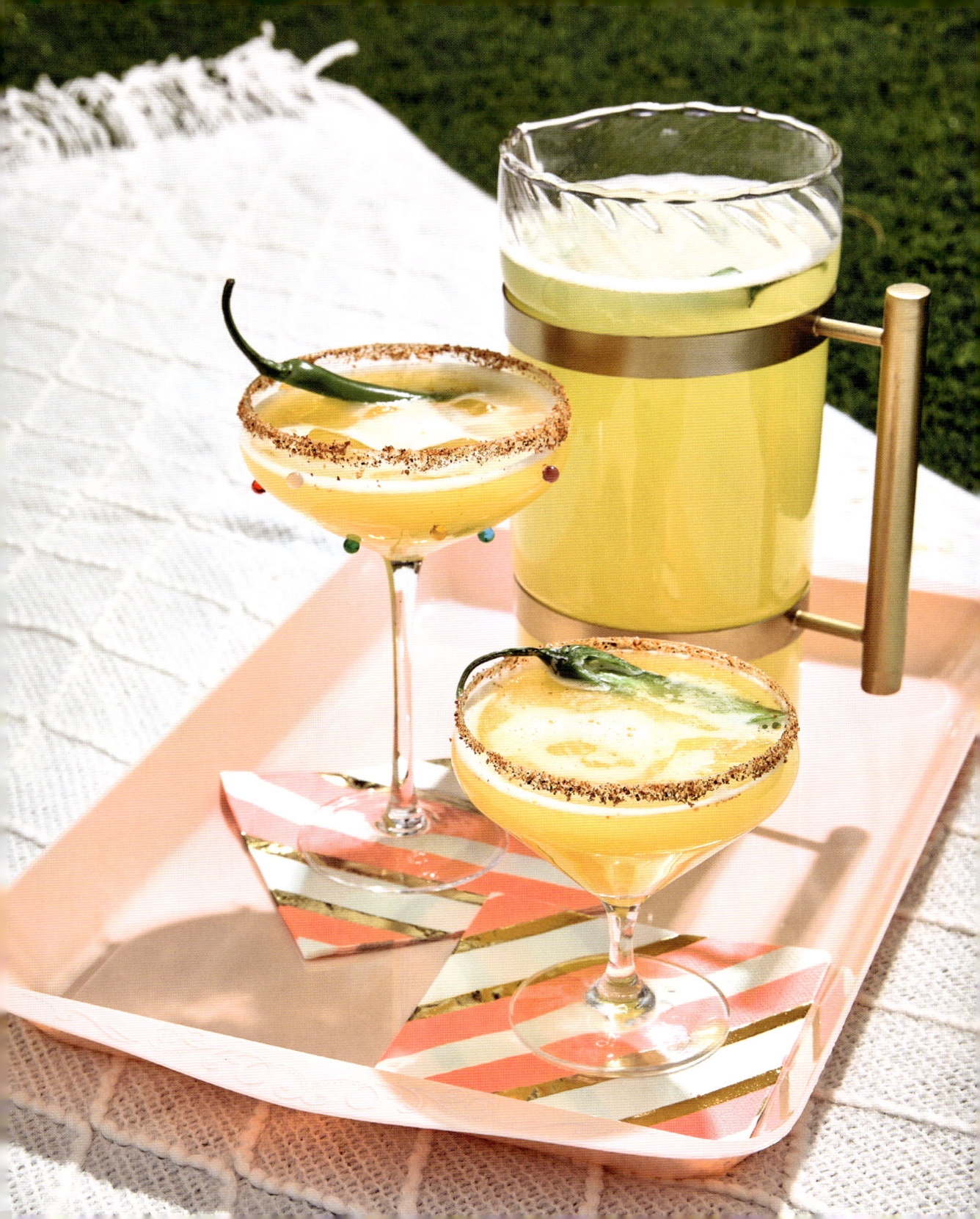

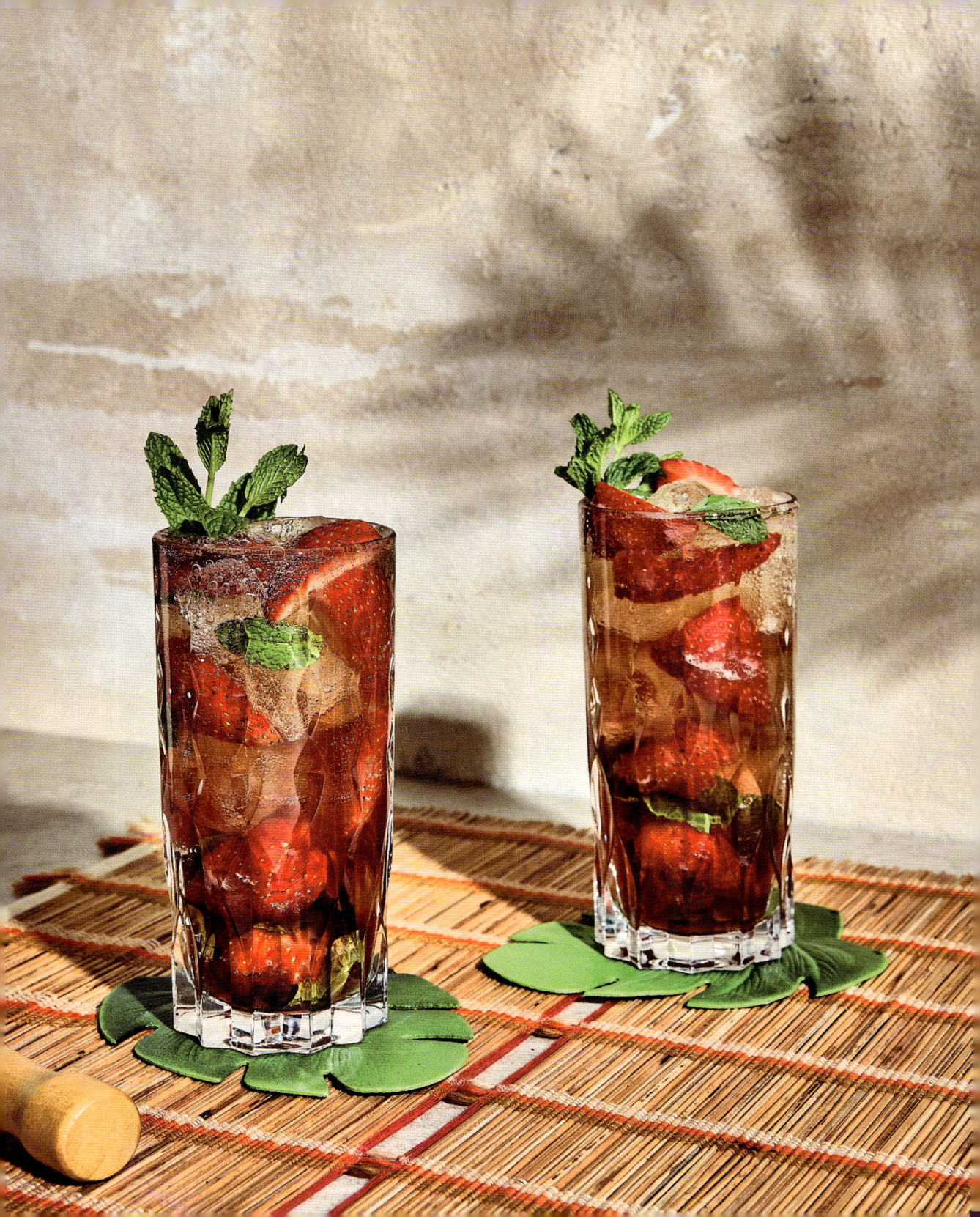

STRAWBERRY POMEGRANATE MOJITO

LIKE A VIRGIN
Mojito

SERVES 1

5 strawberries, cut into thirds (see Tip)

12 mint leaves

2 tablespoons pomegranate juice

Juice of 1 lime

2 teaspoons agave syrup

Ice cubes

1 cup strawberry sparkling water

GARNISH

Strawberry slices

1 mint sprig

1. Place the strawberries in a shaker and muddle them to your liking by gently pressing down and twisting with a muddler or wooden spoon. (I prefer chunks of strawberry, so I muddle 3 to 5 times.)

2. Add the mint leaves, pomegranate juice, lime juice, and agave.

3. Muddle the mint just until you start to smell its aroma (3 to 5 times). Avoid crushing the mint into small pieces. (I like keeping the leaves intact so the mojito is easy to drink and the mint doesn't get caught in the straw.)

4. Add a handful of ice and shake until the outside of the shaker is frosty, about 5 seconds.

5. Open the shaker and pour the entire mixture, ice included, into a tall glass.

6. Add more ice, then top with sparkling water. Stir gently to combine.

7. Garnish with strawberries and mint.

If I knew how good this mojito was going to be, I would've skipped all the years of drinking alcoholic ones and gone straight to these! It's the perfect remix on a classic with juicy strawberry and pomegranate flavors, crisp mint, and the right amount of sass.

TIP Cutting the strawberries into thirds will make them easier to muddle.

Doses & MIMOSAS

SERVES 1

½ cup tangerine juice

Ice cubes

1 tablespoon apple cider vinegar

¼ cup ginger ale

Tangerine wedge, for garnish

1. Combine the tangerine juice and a handful of ice in a shaker. Shake until the outside of the shaker is frosty, about 5 seconds.

2. Strain the tangerine juice into a champagne flute glass.

3. Pour in the apple cider vinegar and stir, then top with ginger ale and a tangerine wedge.

Let's be real: You'll never catch me at a late dinner. But brunch? I will be the first one to RSVP. This is the ultimate bubbly upgrade, a spicy twist on a classic. But fair warning: Now that you have this recipe, you just might start opting for bottomless mimosas at home instead.

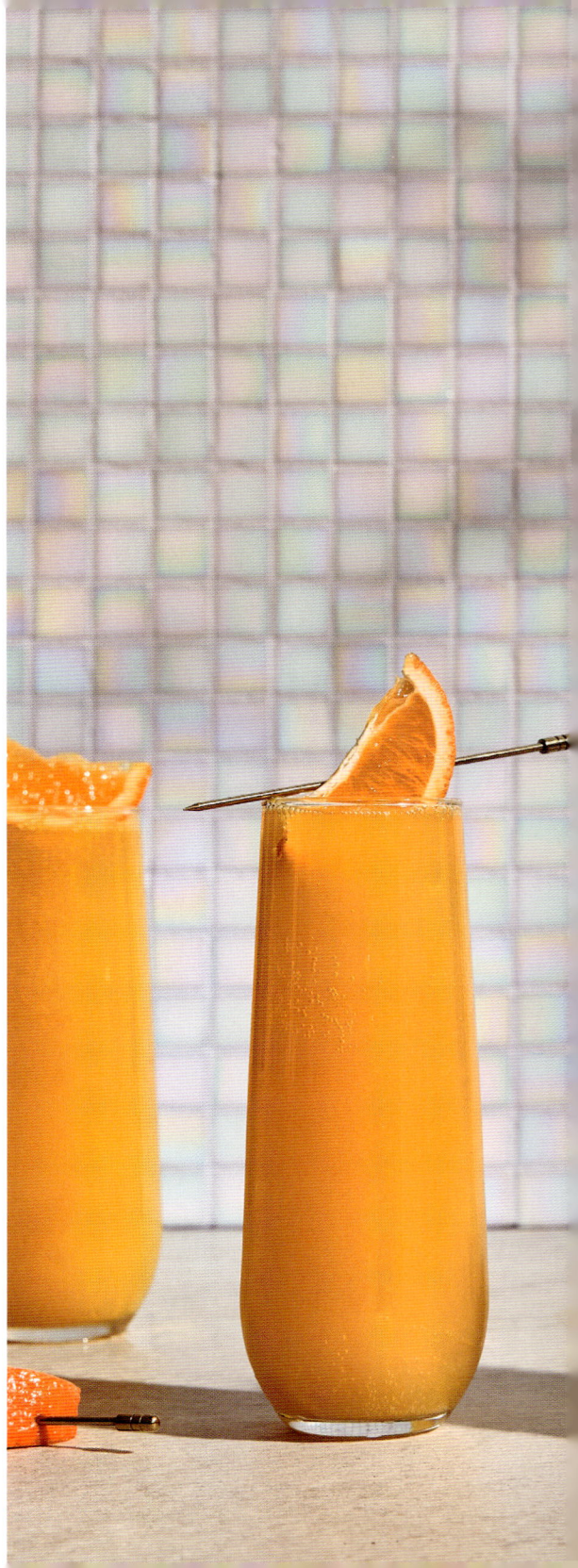

CALL ME MAYBE
Mule

SERVES 1

5 to 7 blackberries, plus extra for garnish

Juice of 1 lime

Ice cubes

1 cup ginger beer, chilled

1. Place the blackberries in a lowball glass and pour in the lime juice.

2. Use a muddler to gently crush the berries, rotating the muddler until the blackberry juice mixes with the lime juice, about 6 twists, or until the blackberries are flattened.

3. Fill the glass with ice, then top with the ginger beer. Stir, add additional blackberries for garnish, and enjoy.

I wanted to make all the recipes in this book super simple and low-lift—because let's be honest, we have things to do and mocktails to drink—and this mule is at the top of the list. A mocktail you can drink and never get sick of, much like the song "Call Me Maybe" by Carly Rae Jepsen. I will never ever get tired of that song!

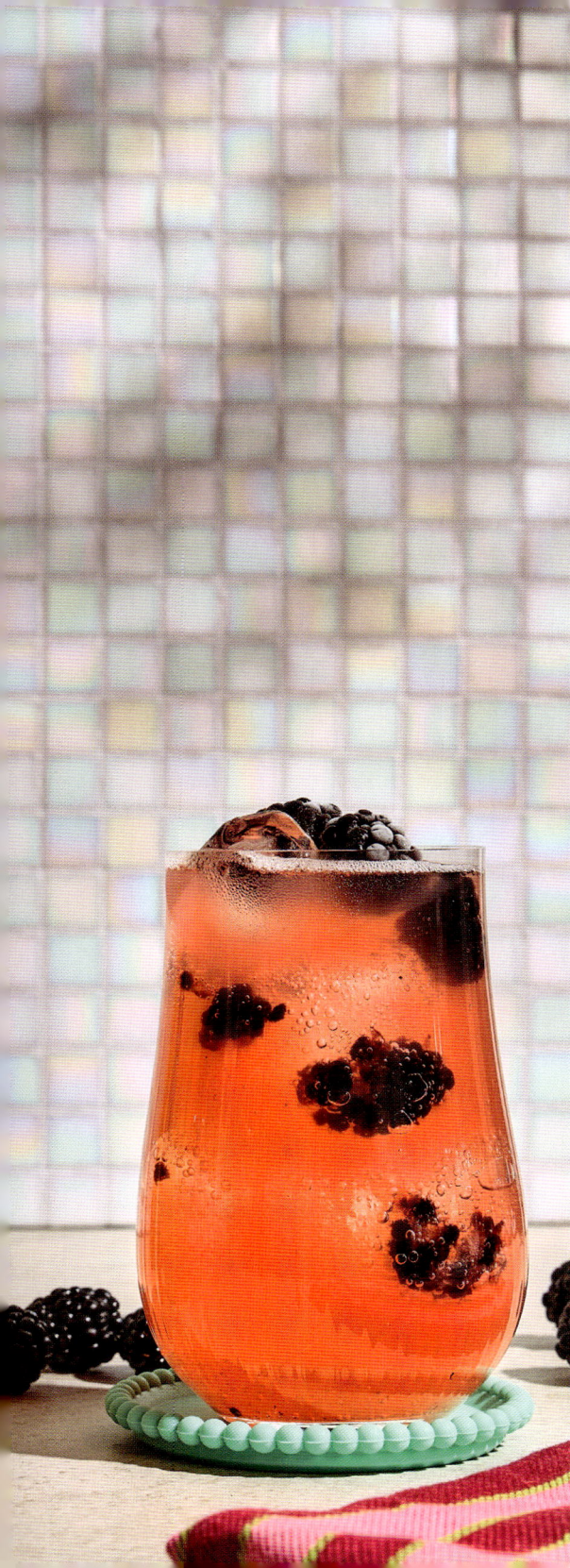

WATERMELON *Sugar*

SERVES 1

1 cup watermelon chunks (5 to 6 big chunks)

¾ cup ice cubes

½ cup lemonade

Juice of 1 lemon

Pinch of salt

Water, if needed

Lemon zest, for garnish (optional)

1. Place the watermelon, ice, lemonade, lemon juice, and salt in a blender.

2. Blend until you reach your desired consistency. Add water if needed.

3. Pour into your favorite wineglass and add lemon zest (if using).

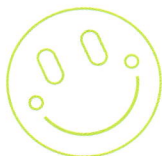

You know the feeling of pure bliss: driving in a car with the windows down, music up, and nothing but good vibes? I remember the summer I made the move back to Florida after 10 years, driving in my car and listening to "Watermelon Sugar" by Harry Styles as the sun was setting. It felt like the perfect soundtrack to a fresh new chapter. That unfiltered joy I experienced is exactly how I want you to feel when sipping on this mocktail. Besides, who doesn't love a frosé?

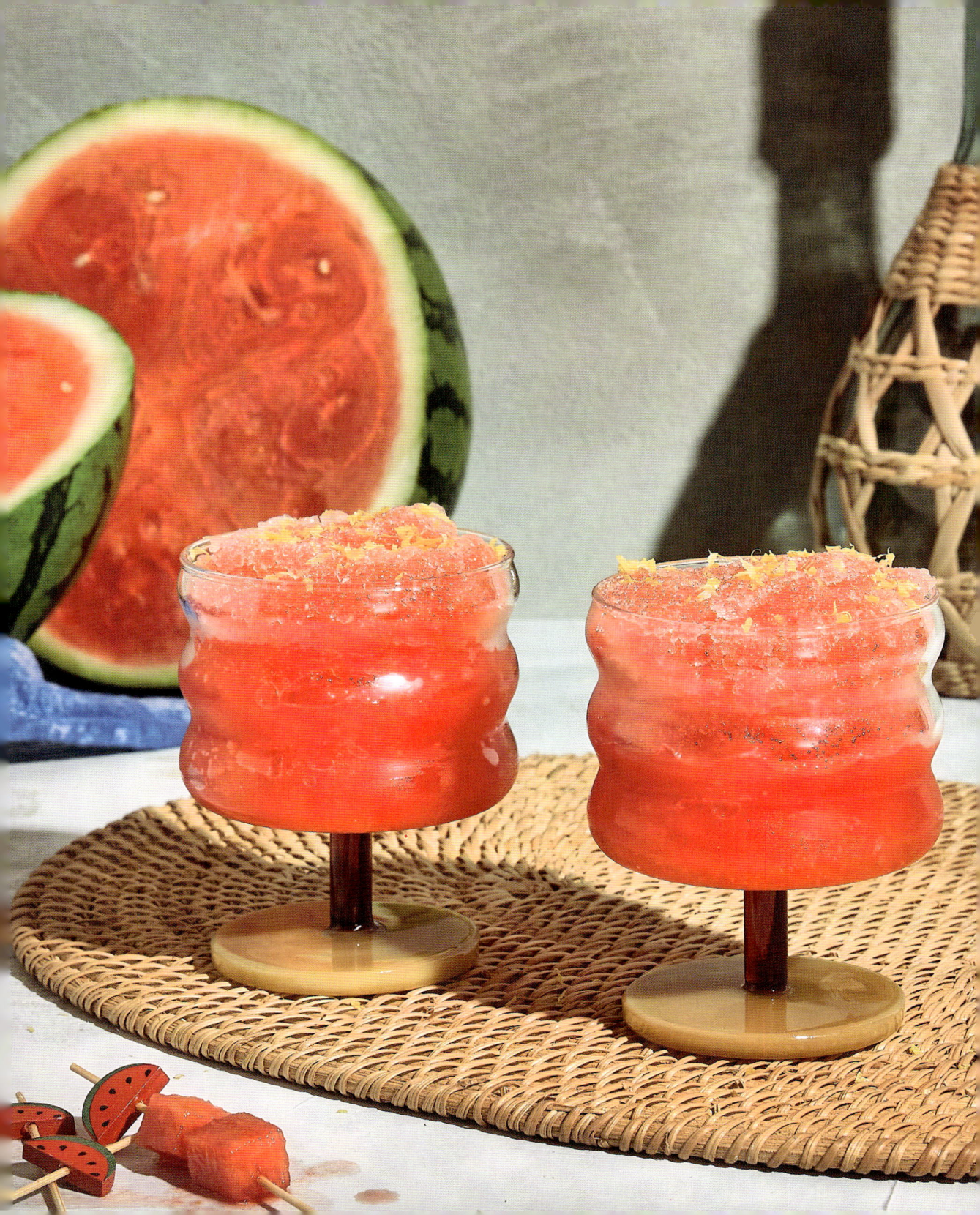

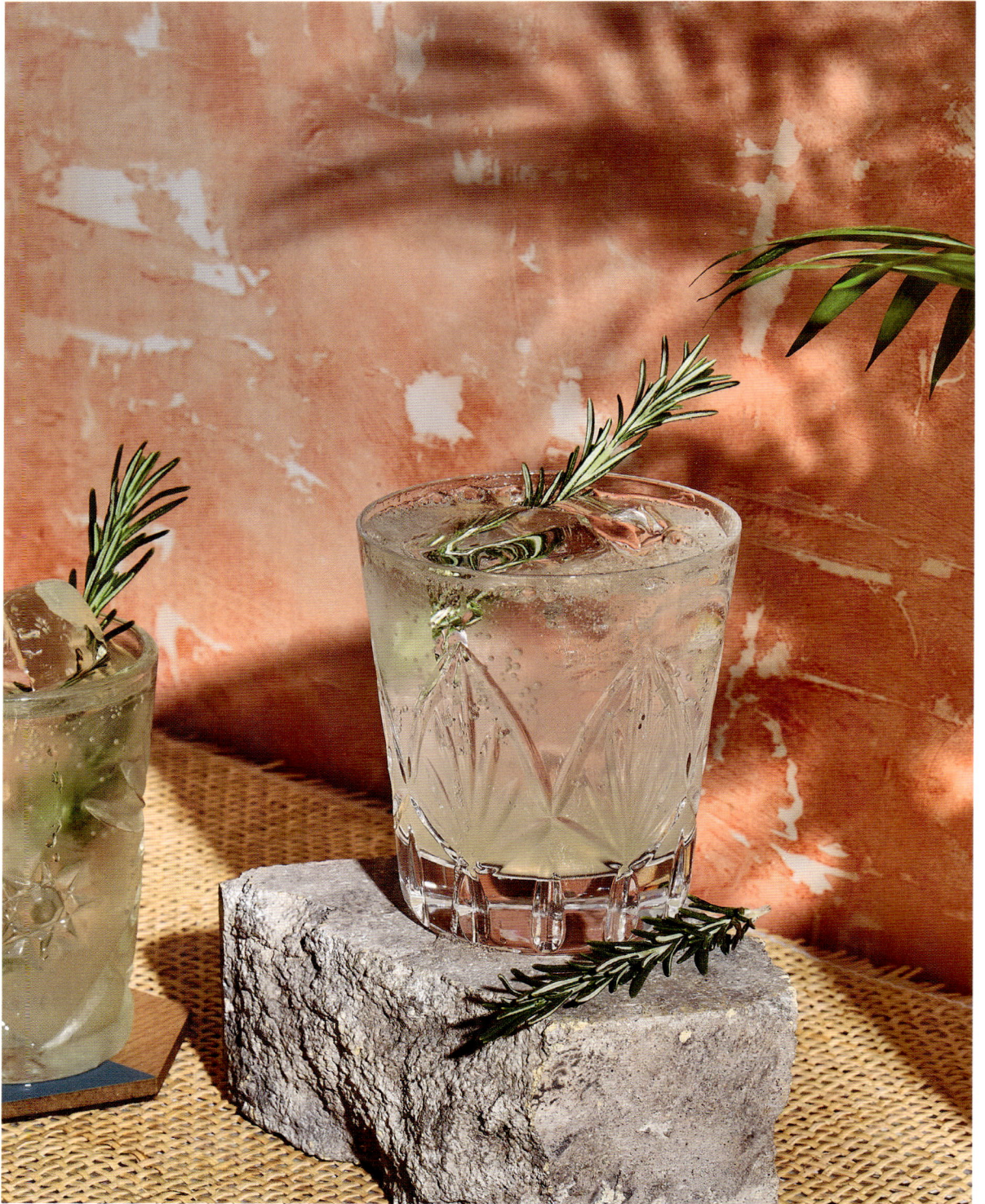

TOXIC *Tonic*

SERVES 1

Juice of ½ lemon

Juice of ½ lime

1 tablespoon elderflower syrup (see Note)

1 rosemary sprig, for garnish

Ice cubes

1 cup elderflower tonic water, chilled (unflavored works, too)

1. Add the lemon juice, lime juice, and elderflower syrup to a highball glass.

2. Use the rosemary sprig to stir.

3. Fill the glass with ice, then pour the tonic water on top.

4. Stir and then garnish with the rosemary sprig.

NOTE Looking to make another mocktail using the elderflower syrup? Try the Garden Cooler (page 113).

A mocktail fit for Queen Britney Spears herself! Years ago, one of my best friends introduced me to gin and tonics with a splash of St. Germain, and when I tell you it became my whole personality, I mean it. After I could no longer stand the taste of tequila, but before I started ordering seltzers-and-lime at weddings, it was the drink I always ordered. It honestly became the only drink I knew how to order. This mocktail version hits the spot without the hangover, so, score!

SAY MY NAME
Spritzer

SERVES 1

¼ cup blueberries

3 to 4 basil leaves

Juice of 1 lemon

1½ teaspoons honey

1 tablespoon apple cider vinegar

Ice cubes

½ cup club soda

GARNISH

Blueberries

1 basil sprig

1. Place the blueberries, basil leaves, lemon juice, and honey in a lowball glass and muddle with a muddler or the back of a wooden spoon until the blueberries break down, 20 to 30 seconds.

2. Add the apple cider vinegar and stir.

3. Fill the glass with ice, then top with club soda.

4. Garnish with additional blueberries and a basil sprig.

TIP To make this drink even more vibrant, simply blend the blueberries, basil, lemon juice, and honey in a blender. Strain into an ice-filled glass, and top with club soda and apple cider vinegar. Stir and enjoy!

This blueberry basil gut-health spritzer will have you feeling all kinds of empowered, much like the classic Destiny's Child song. With the sweet burst of berries, basil aroma, and a gut health–boosting twist, this mocktail will remind you to stand tall, stay true to yourself, and embrace the confidence that comes with taking care of your body.

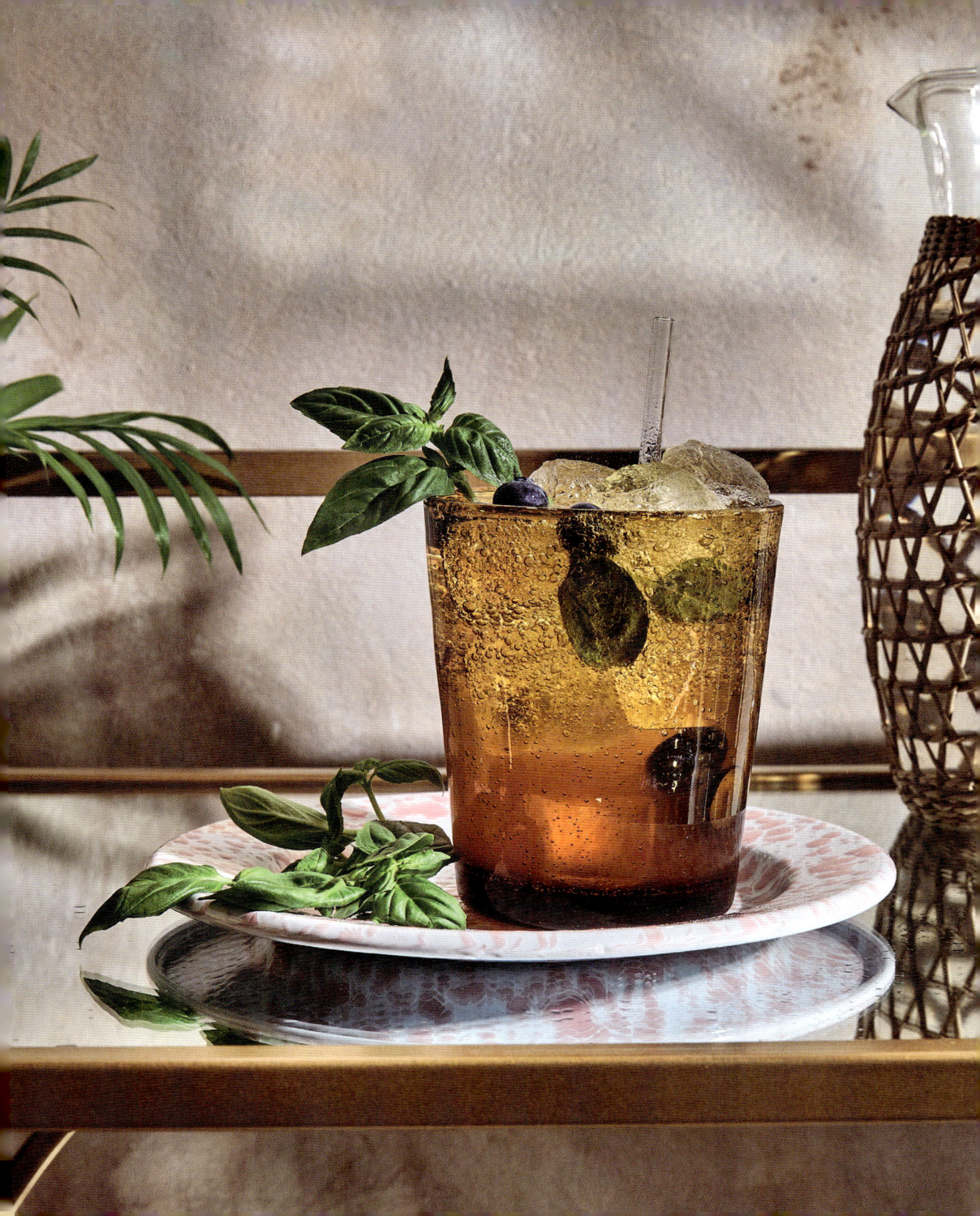

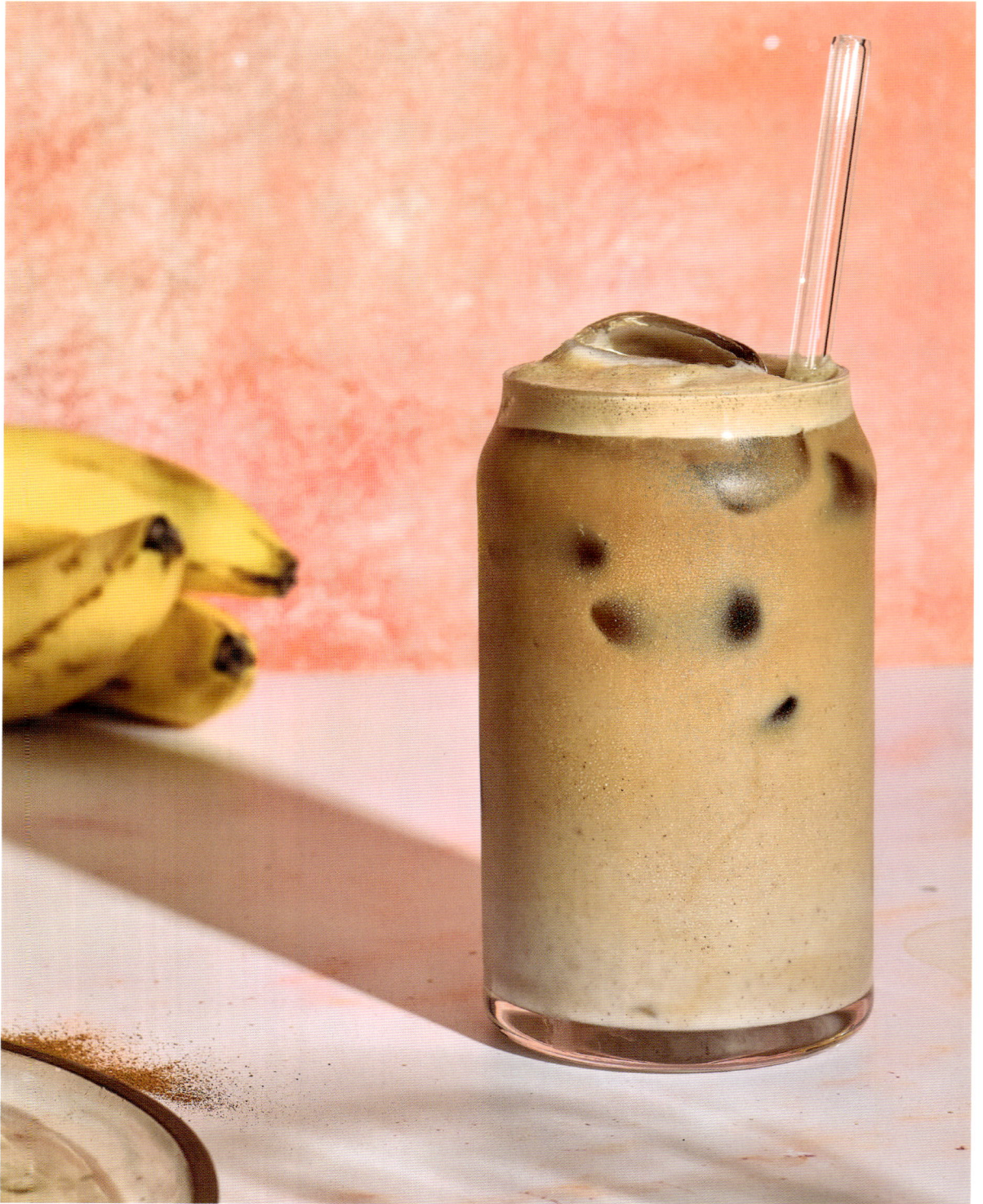

BANANA Montana

SERVES 1

⅓ banana, sliced

⅓ cup oat milk (or milk of choice)

1½ teaspoons agave syrup

Dash of ground cinnamon

Ice cubes

2 shots espresso

1. Place the banana, milk, agave, and cinnamon in a blender and blend until smooth.

2. Fill a tall glass about three-fourths of the way with ice and pour in the banana milk.

3. Top with the espresso. Stir and enjoy!

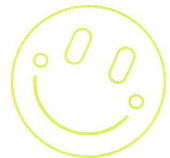

This latte gives you the best of both worlds. Combining the delicious banana bread flavor with the smooth, rich flavors of the espresso creates a perfect balance of cozy and caffeinated. Sweet niblets, this latte is good.

LET'S GO *Girls*

SERVES 1

2 shots espresso (about ½ cup), cooled to room temperature

¼ cup coffee creamer (I like hazelnut)

¼ teaspoon agave syrup, or to taste (depending on the sweetness of your creamer)

¼ teaspoon vanilla extract

Ice cubes

GARNISH

Agave syrup

1½ teaspoons cocoa powder

3 to 5 coffee beans

1. To garnish the rim of your glass, place the agave syrup on a small plate. Place the cocoa powder on another small plate. Roll the rim of a martini glass in the agave, then in the cocoa powder. Set aside.

2. Pour the espresso, coffee creamer, agave, and vanilla into a shaker.

3. Add a handful of ice and shake until the outside of the shaker is frosty, about 5 seconds.

4. Strain the mixture into the martini glass.

5. Garnish with coffee beans and enjoy.

Let's go girls! Because no girls' night out (or in) is complete without an espresso martini. This bold mocktail is as iconic as the lyrics of the song that inspired its name, bringing just the right mix of energy and indulgence. Perfect for toasting to friendship, dancing in the kitchen, or just when you need a little pick-me-up, this one has the power to bring your girls together—one fabulous sip at a time!

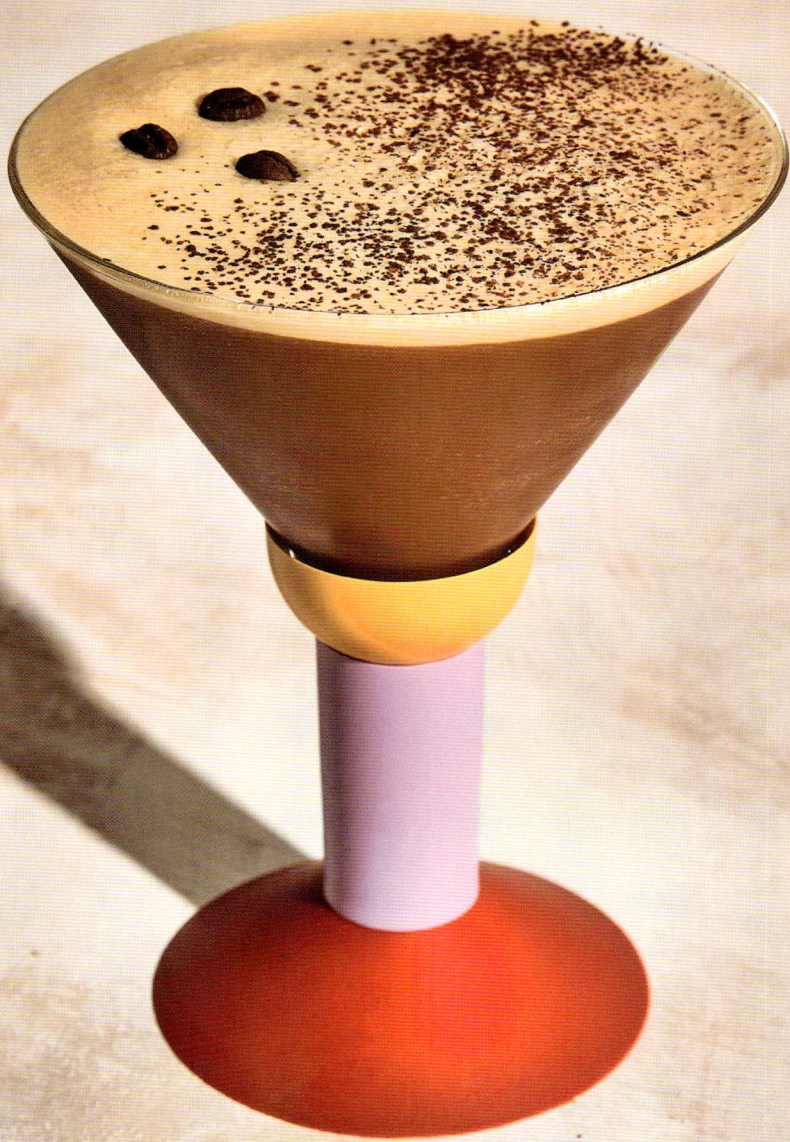

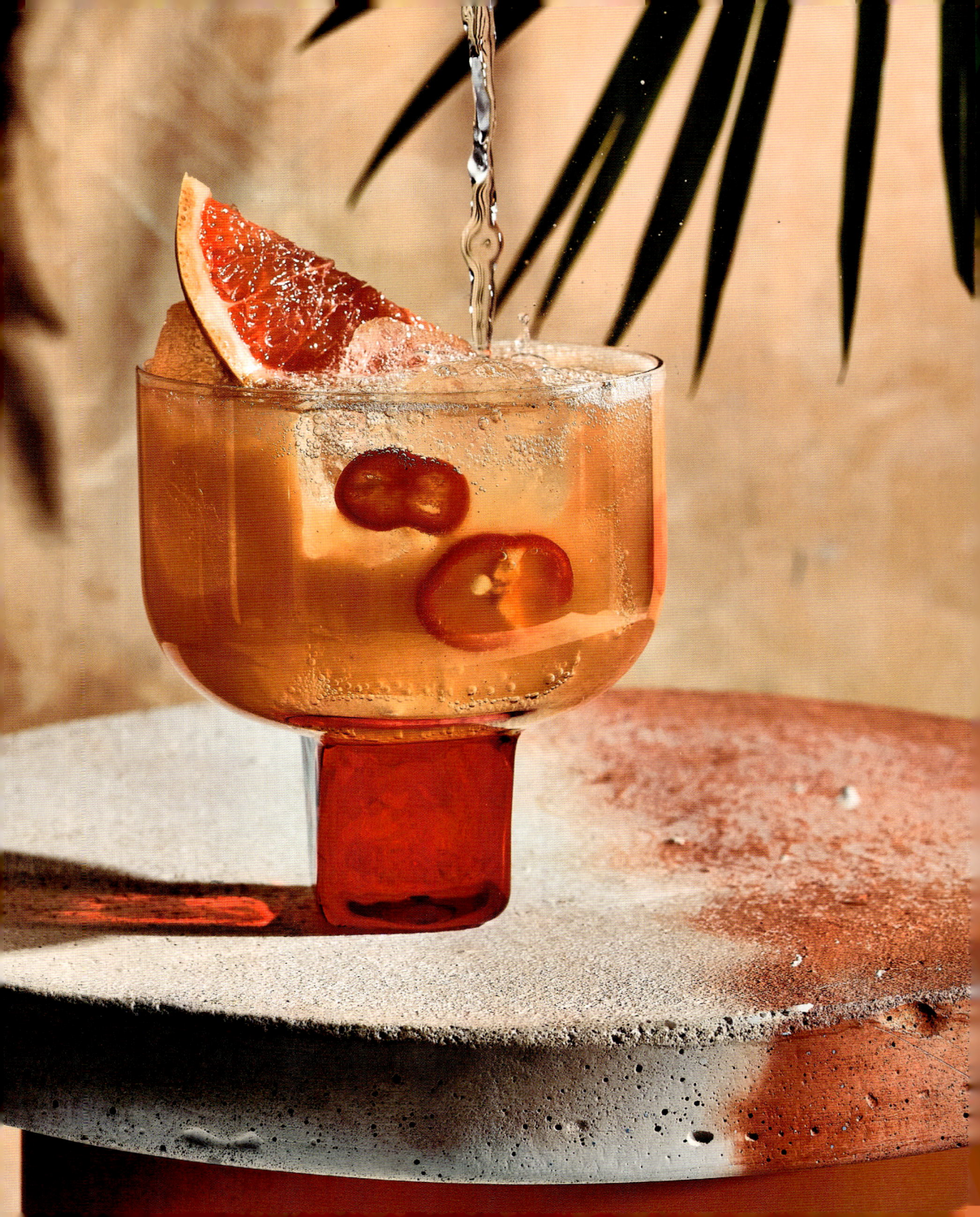

SPICE UP *Your Life*

SERVES 1

Juice of 1½ limes

½ red chile pepper, sliced

½ cup grapefruit juice

Ice cubes

⅓ cup light ginger beer

GARNISH

1 grapefruit slice

Red chile slices (optional)

1. Add the lime juice and red chile slices to a shaker. Use a muddler or the back of a wooden spoon to muddle until the peppers are broken down, 5 to 10 twists.

2. Add the grapefruit juice and a handful of ice.

3. Shake until the outside of the shaker is frosty, about 15 seconds.

4. Fill a lowball glass with ice and strain the mixture into the glass.

5. Top with ginger beer, then garnish with grapefruit and chile slices (if using).

People of the world: Spice up your life! This is the drink for when you're feeling a little extra. With the tart grapefruit, kick of spice, and crisp ginger beer, you'll for sure be channeling Sporty, Scary, Baby, Ginger, or Posh Spice. This drink is all about big vibes, bold flavors, and living your best, spiciest life.

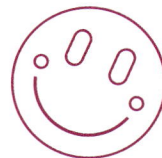

MY FAVORITE MINDFUL
Meditations & Mantras

My thoughts do not control me; I control my thoughts.

I am grateful for the lessons that come with each experience.

I'm allowed to say "no" to protect my energy and time.

I release all expectations and embrace the unknown.

Happiness is within me, waiting for me to choose it.

As I inhale, confidence enters my body. As I exhale, fear exits my body.

I am a work in progress, and I accept that.

I have something of value to give to the world just by being me.

Rather than worry what others think, I choose to live my life for me.

I release negative feelings and choose joy.

Today, I did the best I could. I'm grateful for the effort I was able to give.

My own approval is worth more than the approval of others.

No matter what comes my way, I get to choose how I want to feel and bring my own energy.

I'm grateful to my body for being my home. I commit to taking care of it.

Everything I need is already within me.

Perfection isn't possible. All I expect from myself is to try.

Who I am is exactly who I need to be.

I don't grow by being understood; I grow by understanding myself.

Everything I want is on its way to me.

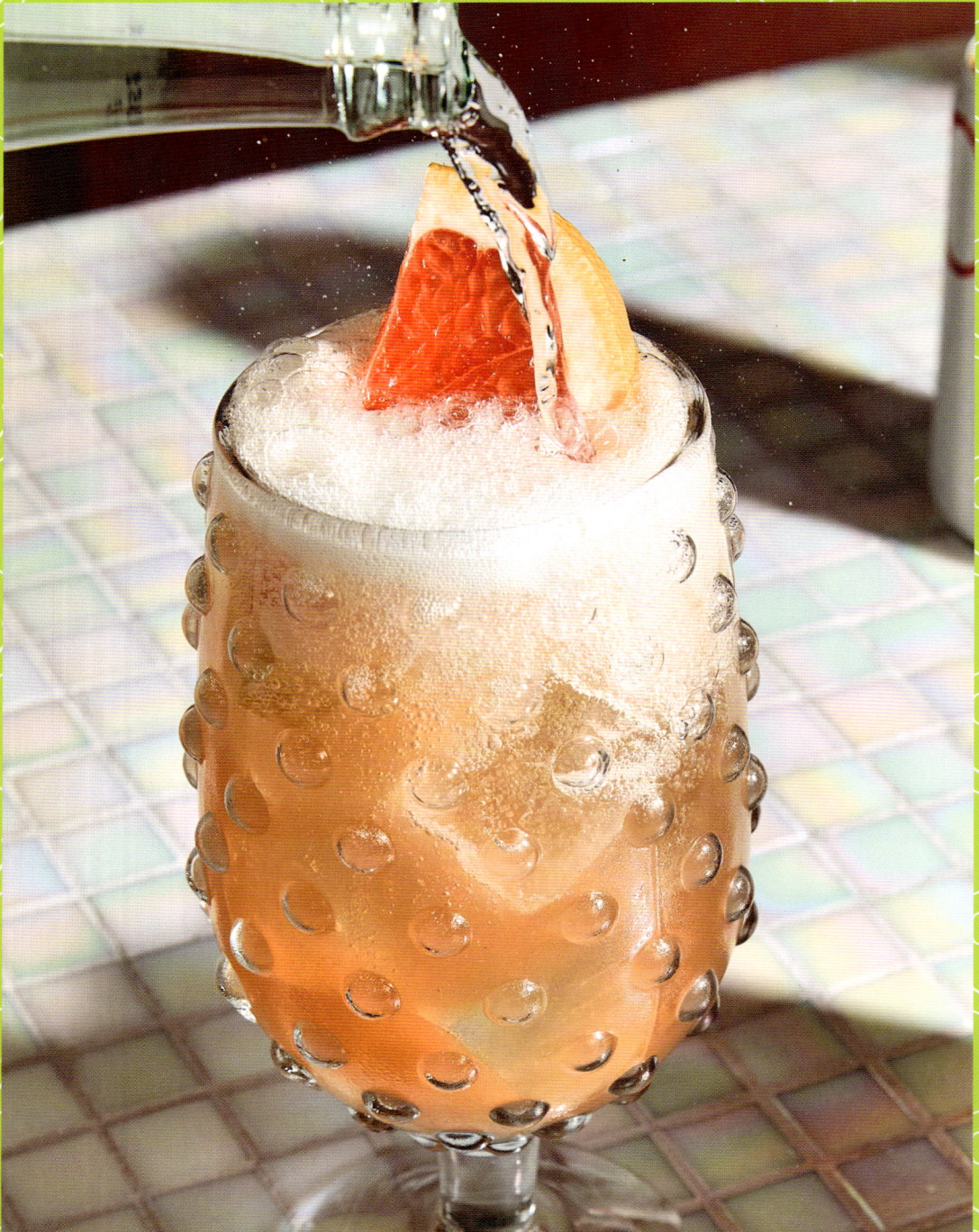

CHAPTER THREE

SELF-CARE
Sips

elf-care comes in many different forms, and sipping on a mocktail from this chapter is my favorite. Ask yourself: *How can I show up for others when I can't even show up for myself?* Remember, self-care is never selfish.

TART CHERRY BEDTIME JUICE

SLEEPY GIRL
Mocktail

SERVES 1

Juice of 1 lime

2 rosemary sprigs, divided

⅓ teaspoon grated ginger

½ cup tart cherry juice

Ice cubes

½ cup sparkling water (flavor of your choosing)

1. Place the lime juice, 1 rosemary sprig, and the ginger in a shaker. Muddle with a muddler or the back of a wooden spoon until the rosemary releases its fragrance and the ginger is worked into the lime juice, 5 to 8 twists.

2. Add the tart cherry juice and a handful of ice. Shake until the outside of the shaker is frosty, about 5 seconds.

3. Fill a lowball glass with ice.

4. Strain the cherry mixture over the ice and top with the sparkling water. Garnish with the remaining rosemary sprig.

This Sleepy Girl Mocktail is my version of red wine. I make this drink as a nightcap, on holidays, and even on a random Tuesday while watching my shows (and on special occasions, I sometimes add a little edible glitter). It's actually a drink my husband craves weekly. Tart cherry juice is great for muscle recovery and helps improve sleep quality, which has been lacking since I became a mom. Sometimes I'll mix in some magnesium as well for some extra relaxation.

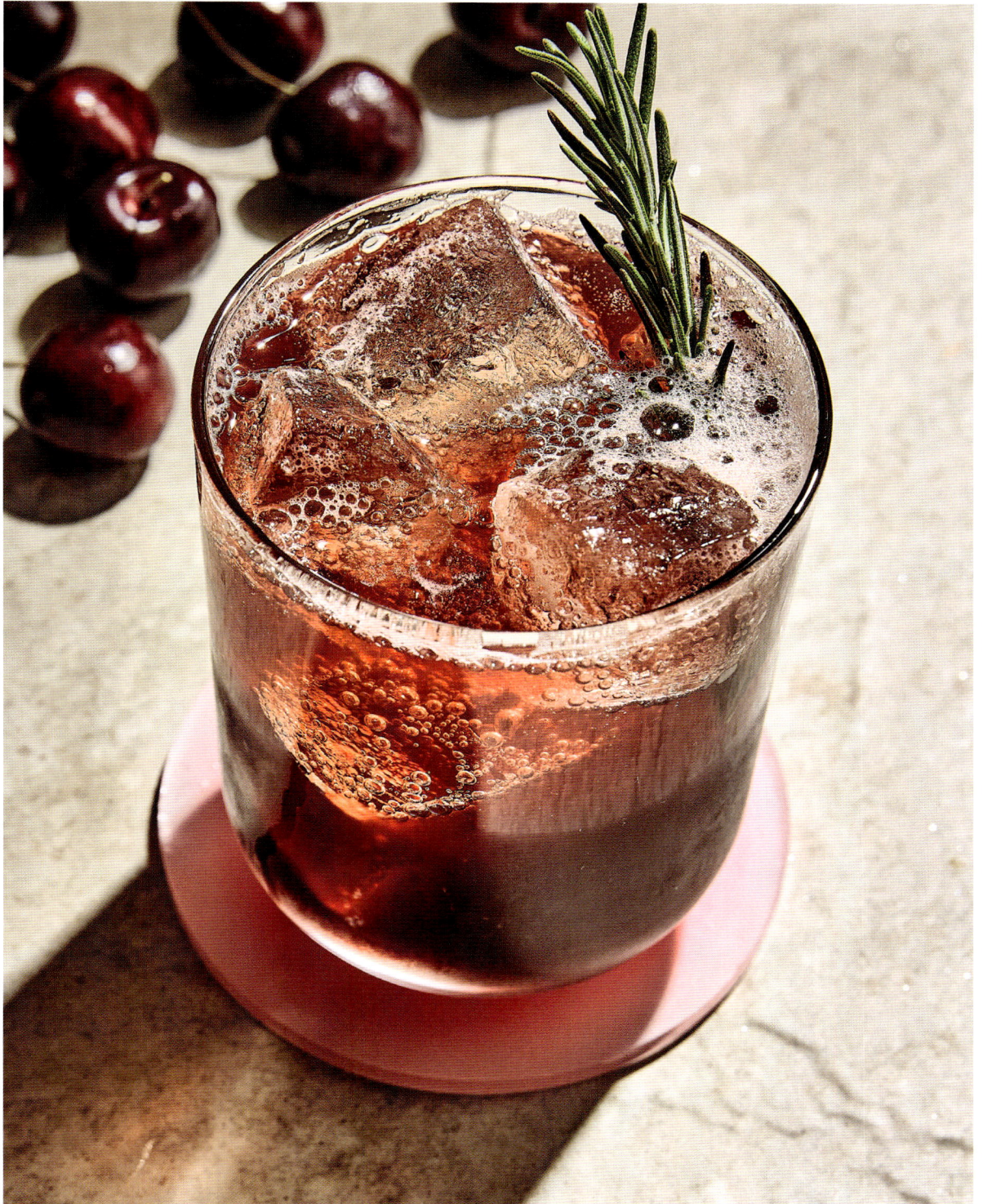

TASTES LIKE *Nostalgia*

SERVES 1

1 cup cereal of choice (I like Magic Spoon's Fruity flavor)

1 cup milk of choice

Ice cubes

2 shots espresso, cooled to room temperature

Handful of cereal pieces, for garnish

1. Add the cereal and milk to a blender. Blend until the cereal dissolves into the milk.

2. Fill a tall glass with ice.

3. Use a fine-mesh strainer to strain the milk mixture into the glass.

4. Top with the espresso, stir, and then garnish with the cereal pieces.

Tastes Like Nostalgia is basically my childhood in a cup. It's the sweet, creamy last sips of cereal-milk magic, now all grown up with a shot of espresso to keep you functioning like an actual adult. One sip and suddenly you're back in your pj's, parked in front of the TV, watching The Fairly OddParents. *Whether you were a Froot Loops kid or a Cinnamon Toast Crunch ride-or-die, this latte brings all those childhood vibes back, with a little caffeine to keep you going.*

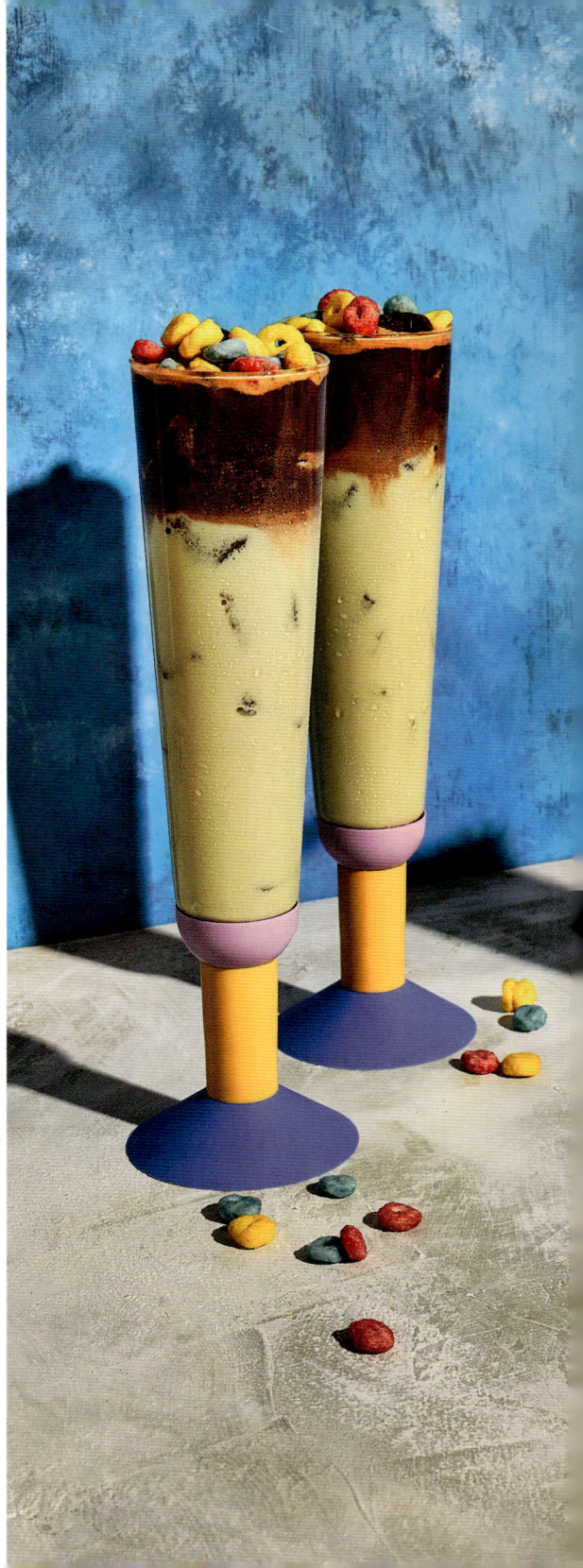

ICED COCONUT PASSION FRUIT TEA

TREAT YOURSELF
Tea

SERVES 1

¾ cup boiling water

1 passion fruit tea bag

½ cup coconut milk

2 tablespoons white grape juice

1½ tablespoons agave syrup

3 to 5 frozen strawberries (optional)

Ice cubes

1. Steep the tea bag in the boiling water for 5 to 7 minutes. Remove the tea bag and set the tea aside to cool to room temperature.

2. Add the coconut milk, grape juice, agave, and strawberries (if using) to a highball glass. Stir for about 10 seconds.

3. Add 1 to 2 handfuls of ice (I prefer 2) to your glass, then top with the tea.

4. Gently stir and enjoy!

Some days you just need to treat yourself, and this drink delivers! The creamy coconut mixed with the tangy passion fruit tea gives you a smooth sip every time, reminding you that it's important to pause, relax, and treat yourself when you need it.

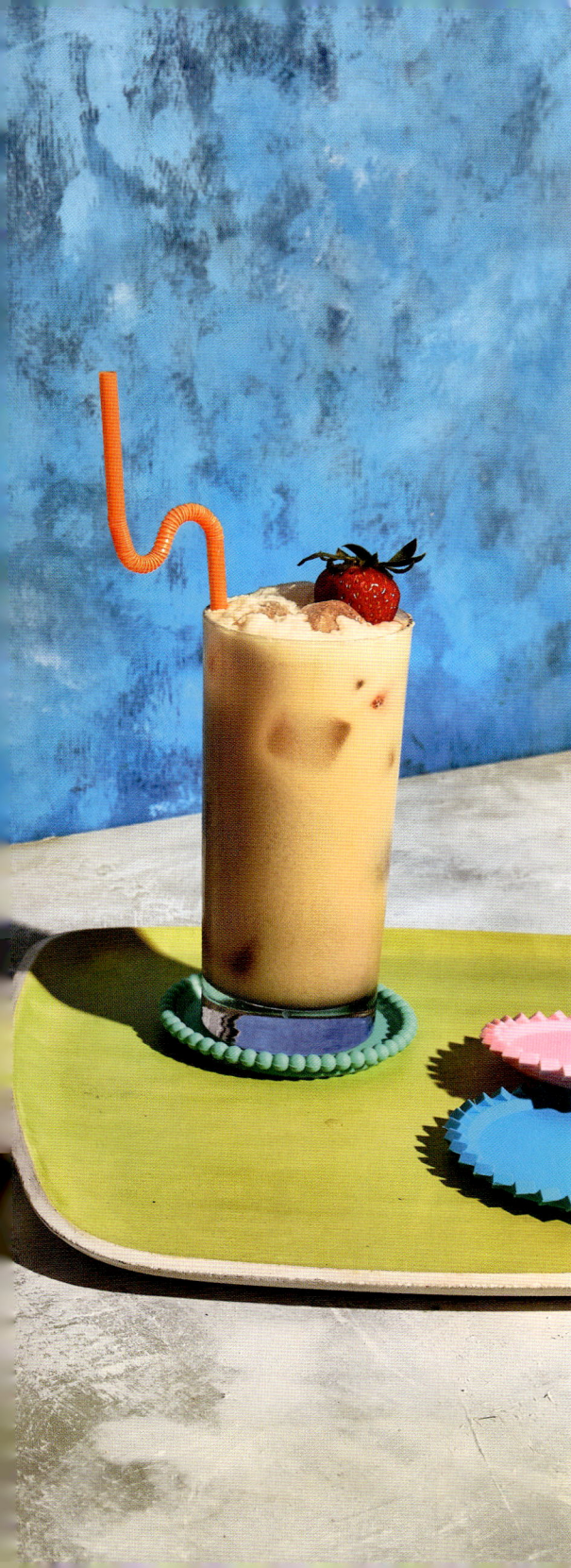

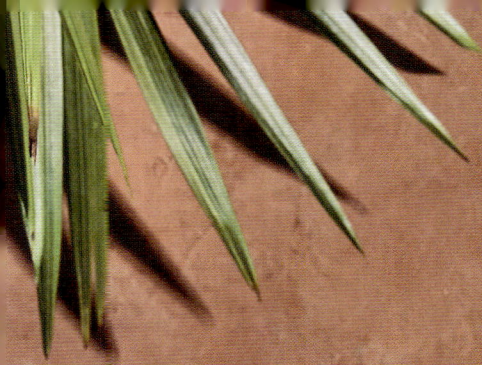

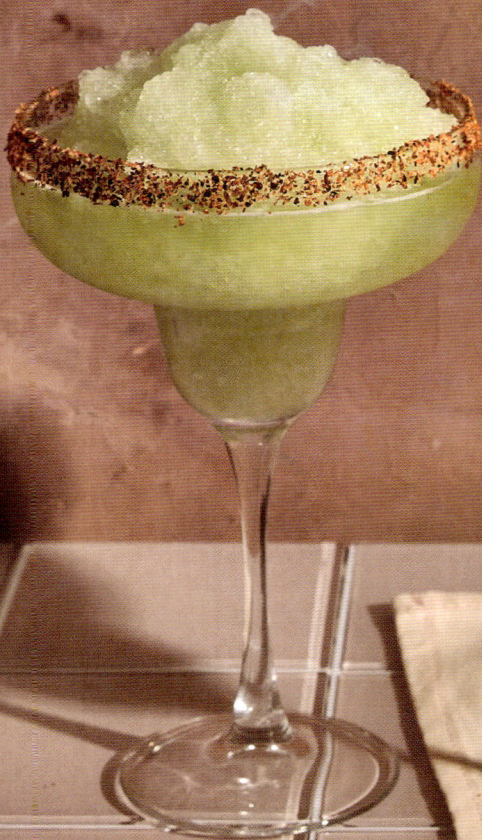

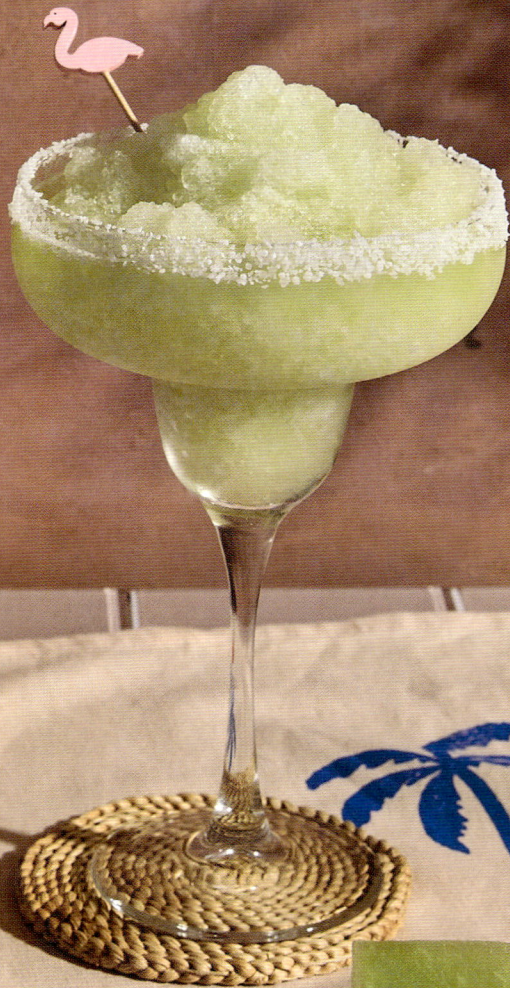

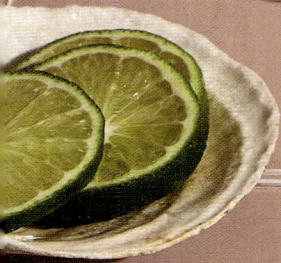

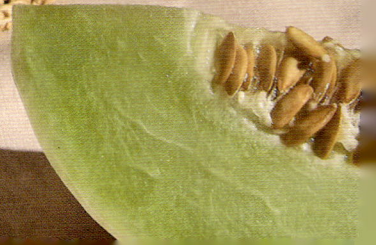

YOU DEW *You*

SERVES 1

5 or 6 big honeydew melon chunks (about 1 cup)

1 cup ice

¼ cup water (optional, if needed)

Juice of 1 small lemon

2 tablespoons orange juice

2 tablespoons pineapple juice

1. Place all the ingredients into a blender and blend until slushy.

2. Pour the mixture into a margarita glass and enjoy.

NOTE Want some spice? Rub a lemon wedge around the rim of your glass and roll it in Tajín, then pour the margarita into the glass.

If you're into tennis or even if you're not, I guarantee you have heard of the Honey Deuce, the popular drink that is the talk of the town every August when the US Open rolls around. I figured we needed a Callie mocktail version of it that is going to serve (hehe). Fun fact: One of my sisters won the US Open for mixed doubles, and I was there to witness it. I also got to meet Roger Federer and shake his hand, so as you can expect, the US Open holds a special place in my heart.

SO FETCH
Spritz

SERVES 1

½ cup grapefruit juice

Juice of ½ lime

2 teaspoons lavender syrup

1 teaspoon agave syrup

Ice cubes

½ cup grapefruit sparkling water

1 grapefruit slice, for garnish

1. Place the grapefruit juice, lime juice, lavender syrup, and agave in a shaker.

2. Add a handful of ice and shake until the outside of the shaker is frosty, about 5 seconds.

3. Fill a stemmed glass with ice. Strain the grapefruit mixture into the glass.

4. Top with sparkling water and garnish with a grapefruit slice.

Good news: You can sit (sip) with us! The So Fetch Spritz is here to bring the fun with grapefruit and lavender vibes that are as iconic as army pants and flip-flops. Gretchen would be so happy that we're making "fetch" happen. If you like this drink, check out the Lavender Haze Punch (page 128), which also uses lavender syrup.

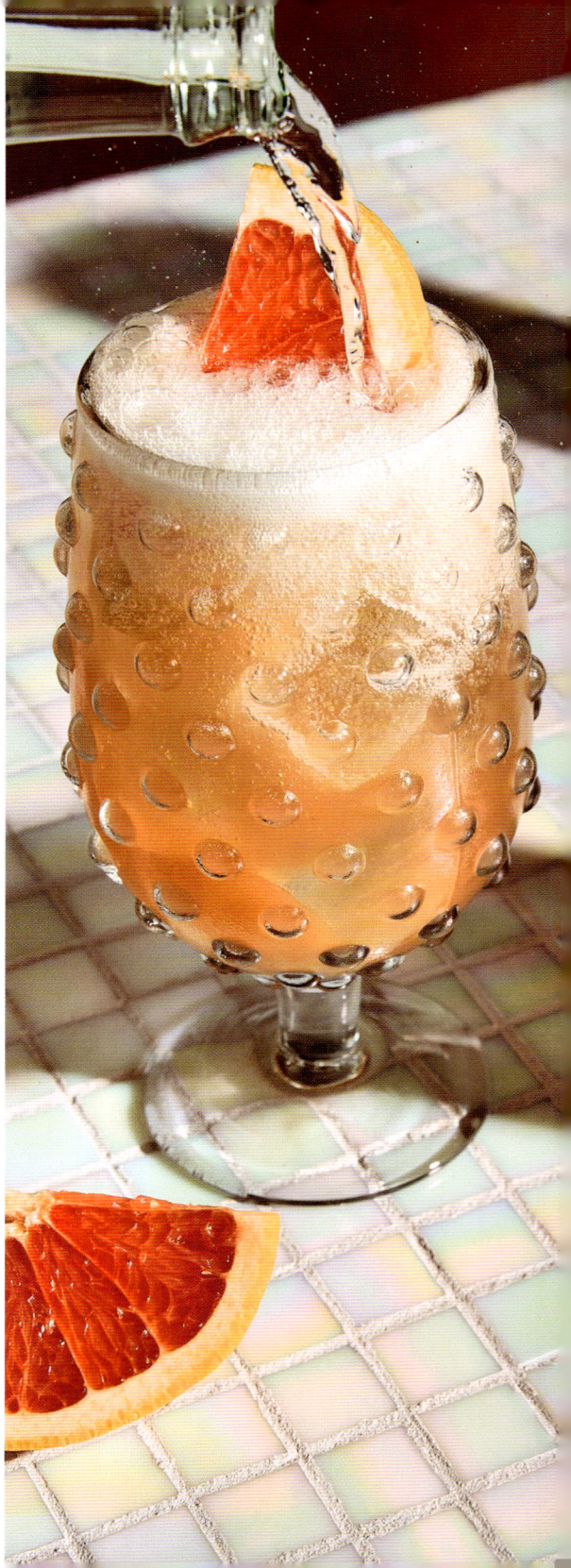

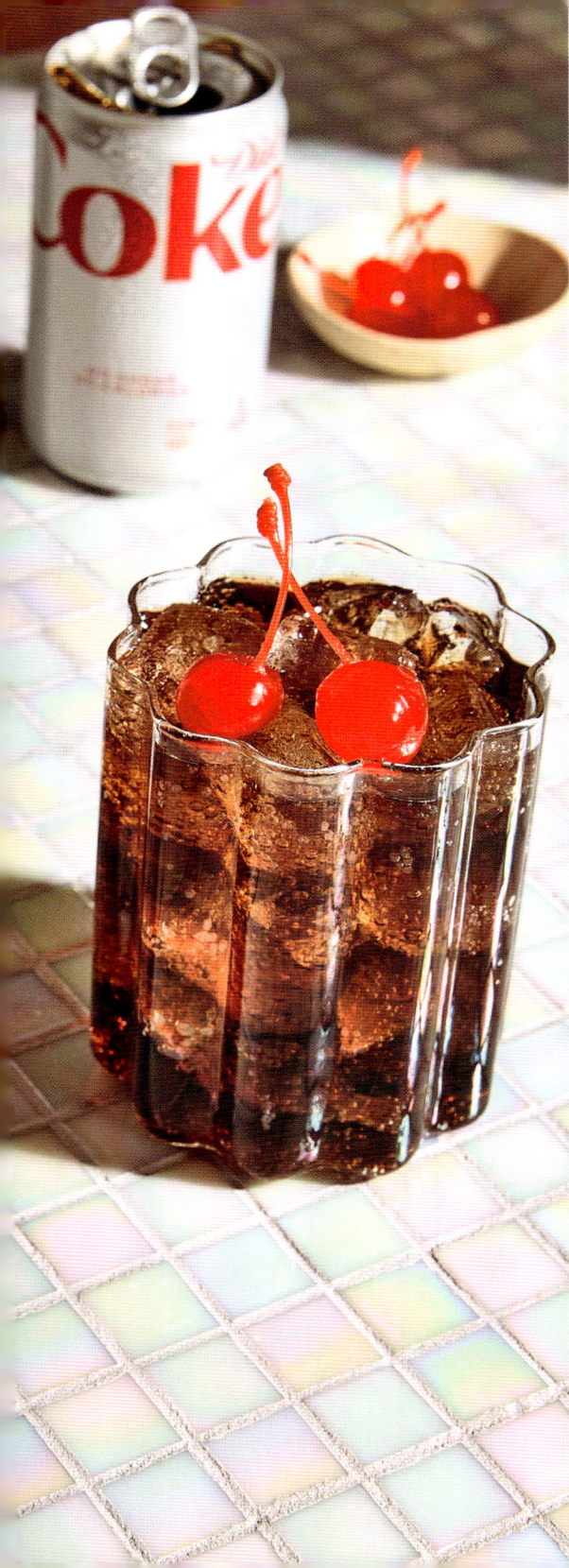

DIRTY POP

SERVES 1

Ice cubes

1 cup Diet Coke

Juice of ½ lime

1 tablespoon grenadine or maraschino cherry juice

Maraschino cherries, for garnish

1. Fill a lowball glass with ice. Pour in the Diet Coke.

2. Add the lime juice and grenadine.

3. Stir and garnish with cherries.

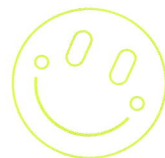

This mocktail is just as irresistible as an early 2000s pop song. The cold, crisp Diet Coke with a little grenadine makes this drink a retro twist on a Shirley Temple, throwing it back to the good ol' times. Dirty Pop is sure to bring the flavor and the vibe.

CHILL WITH *Dill*

SERVES 1

¼ cup pickle juice, from a pickle jar (I like Wickles Pickles, because it's sweet and spicy)

Juice of 1 lime

½ tablespoon agave syrup

Ice cubes

½ cup unflavored sparkling water

GARNISH

½ teaspoon agave syrup

1 teaspoon Tajín

1 teaspoon salt

2 small pickles

1. To garnish the rim of your glass, add ½ teaspoon agave to a small plate. Mix the Tajín and salt on another small plate. Roll the rim of a rocks glass in the agave, then dip it into the Tajín and salt.

2. Add the pickle juice, lime juice, agave, and a handful of ice to a shaker.

3. Shake until the outside of the shaker is frosty, about 15 seconds.

4. Fill the glass with ice, then strain the juice mixture into the glass.

5. Top with sparkling water and garnish with pickles.

Pickles were basically my lifeline during pregnancy, so Chill with Dill is a margarita after my own heart. This pickleback combined with a refreshing marg is salty, tangy, and briny, a true reminder that you can do both. It's unexpected, but let me tell you, it works.

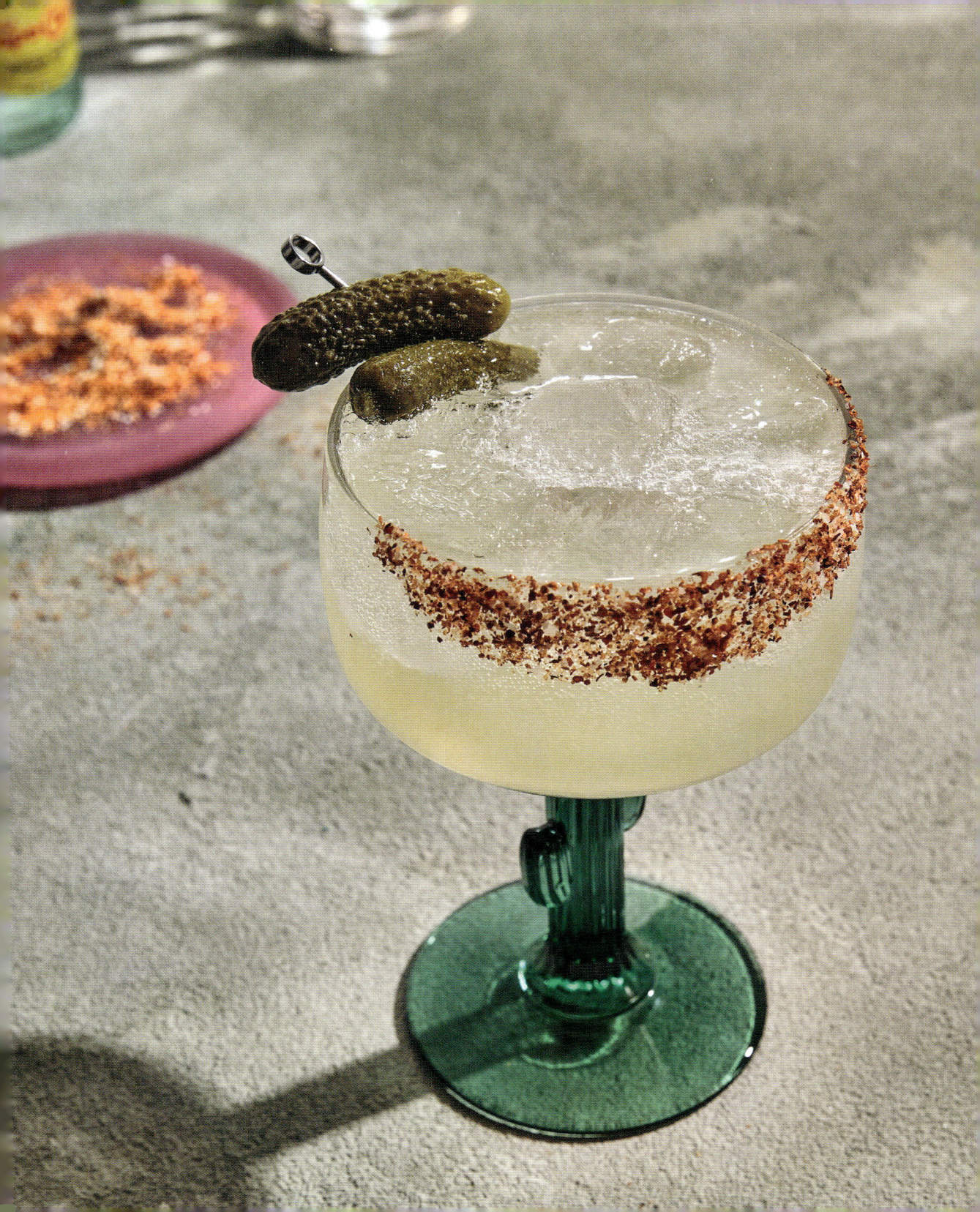

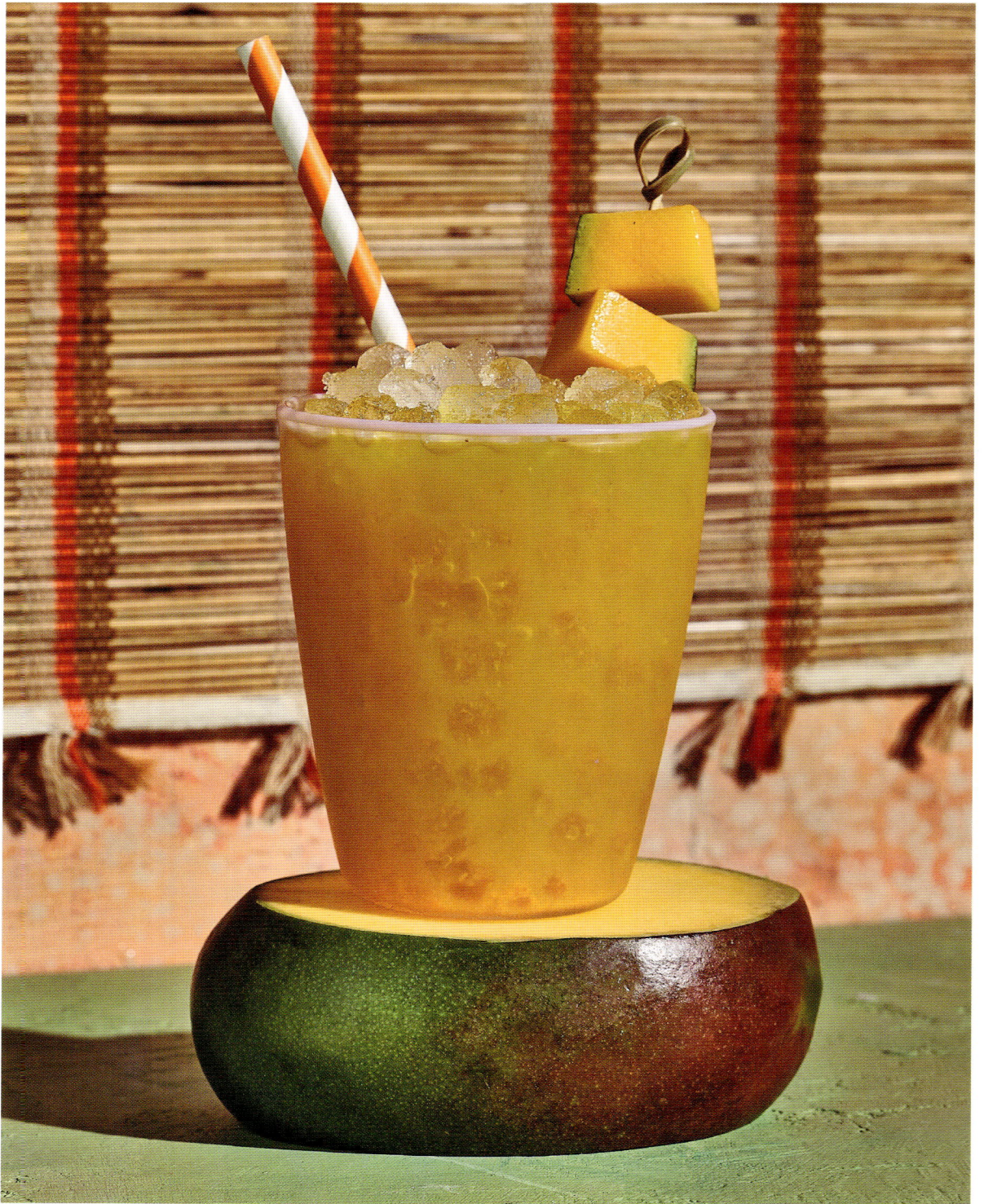

STAY GOLDEN

SERVES 1

¼ cup mango juice

¼ cup coconut water

Juice of ½ lemon

¼ teaspoon grated ginger

¼ teaspoon ground turmeric

Pinch of black pepper (optional, to enhance turmeric absorption)

Ice cubes

1. Combine the mango juice, coconut water, lemon juice, ginger, turmeric, and black pepper (if using) in a shaker. Give it a nice stir.

2. Add a handful of ice and shake until the outside of the shaker is frosty, about 5 seconds.

3. Fill a lowball glass with ice, strain the juice mixture into the glass, and enjoy.

TIP I used to buy mango juice from the juice aisle in the grocery store, and I sometimes still do, but my life was forever changed when my neighbor brought us fresh mangos from his tree. To make your own mango juice without a juicer, blend ½ mango and ⅓ cup water in a blender, then strain through a cheesecloth or mesh strainer.

This is the ultimate refresher. It blends sweet mango and earthy turmeric, which makes it just as delicious as it is nourishing. Adding black pepper helps your body absorb turmeric more effectively, boosting its anti-inflammatory and antioxidant benefits. A drink this zesty and uplifting proves that staying golden isn't just a mindset: It's a lifestyle. If you like this one, you'll love The Detox (page 158) and Forever Young (page 131) shots.

WARM VANILLA CHAMOMILE TEA
CALMING *Creamer*

SERVES 1

˝½ cups milk of choice

2 chamomile tea bags

˝ to 2 tablespoons honey, to taste

˝ teaspoon vanilla extract

Dash of ground cinnamon, for garnish (optional)

1. Heat the milk in a small saucepan over medium heat until it starts to steam, about 4 minutes.

2. Add the tea bags and remove the pan from the heat. Do not let it boil.

3. Steep for 5 to 7 minutes, stirring occasionally.

4. Strain into a mug then add the honey and vanilla. Froth using a frother, if desired.

5. Sprinkle with cinnamon (if using) and enjoy.

ICED CALMING CREAMER
Want it iced? Add the honey and vanilla to the milk and tea mixture. Set aside to cool, then pour over ice.

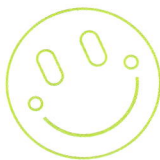

Sometimes you need a cozy moment to yourself—a warm hug in a glass. Nothing beats making this tea, putting on comfies, and relaxing with a romance novel in hand. Whether you're enjoying it on a slow morning or a quiet evening, this sip is pure comfort.

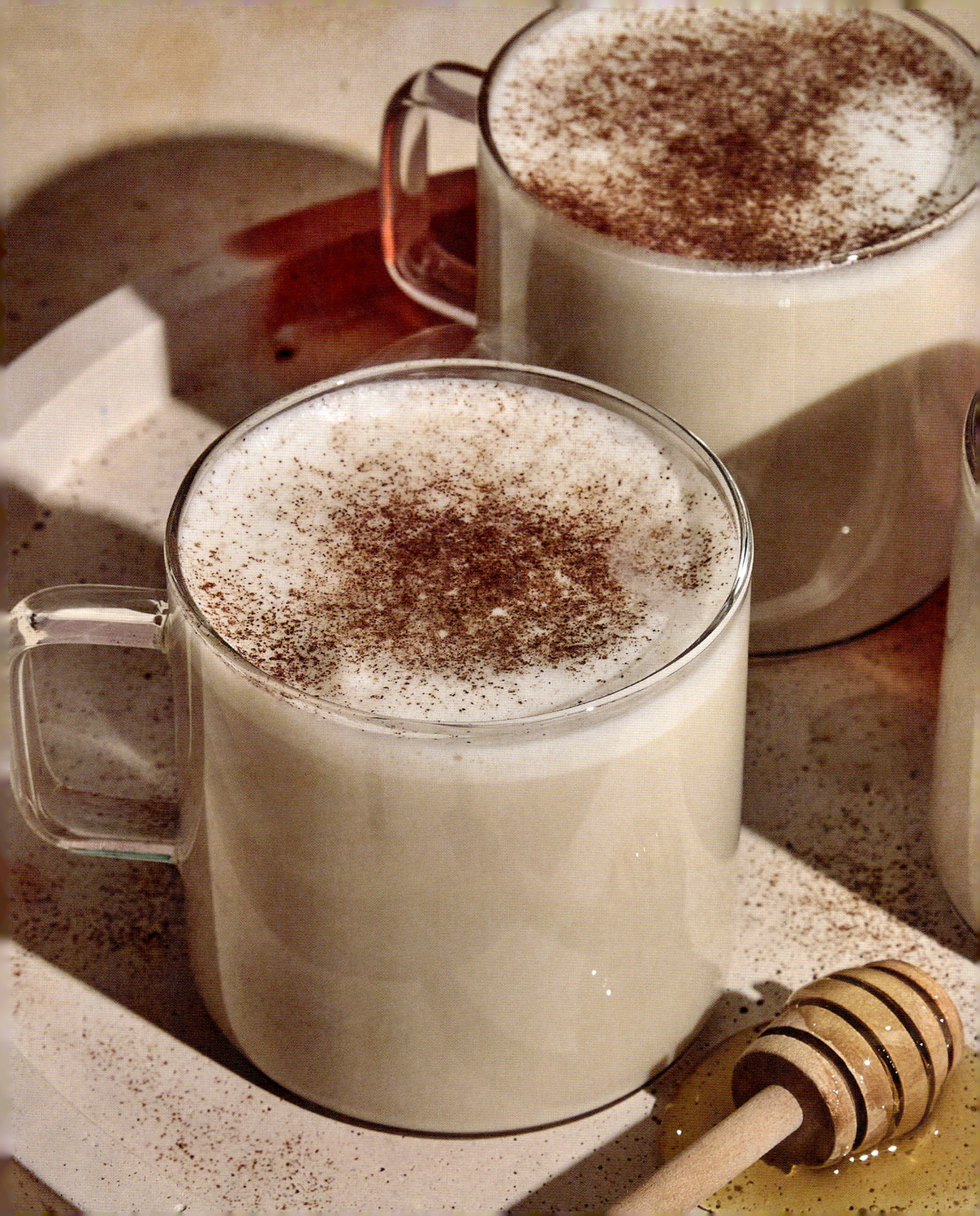

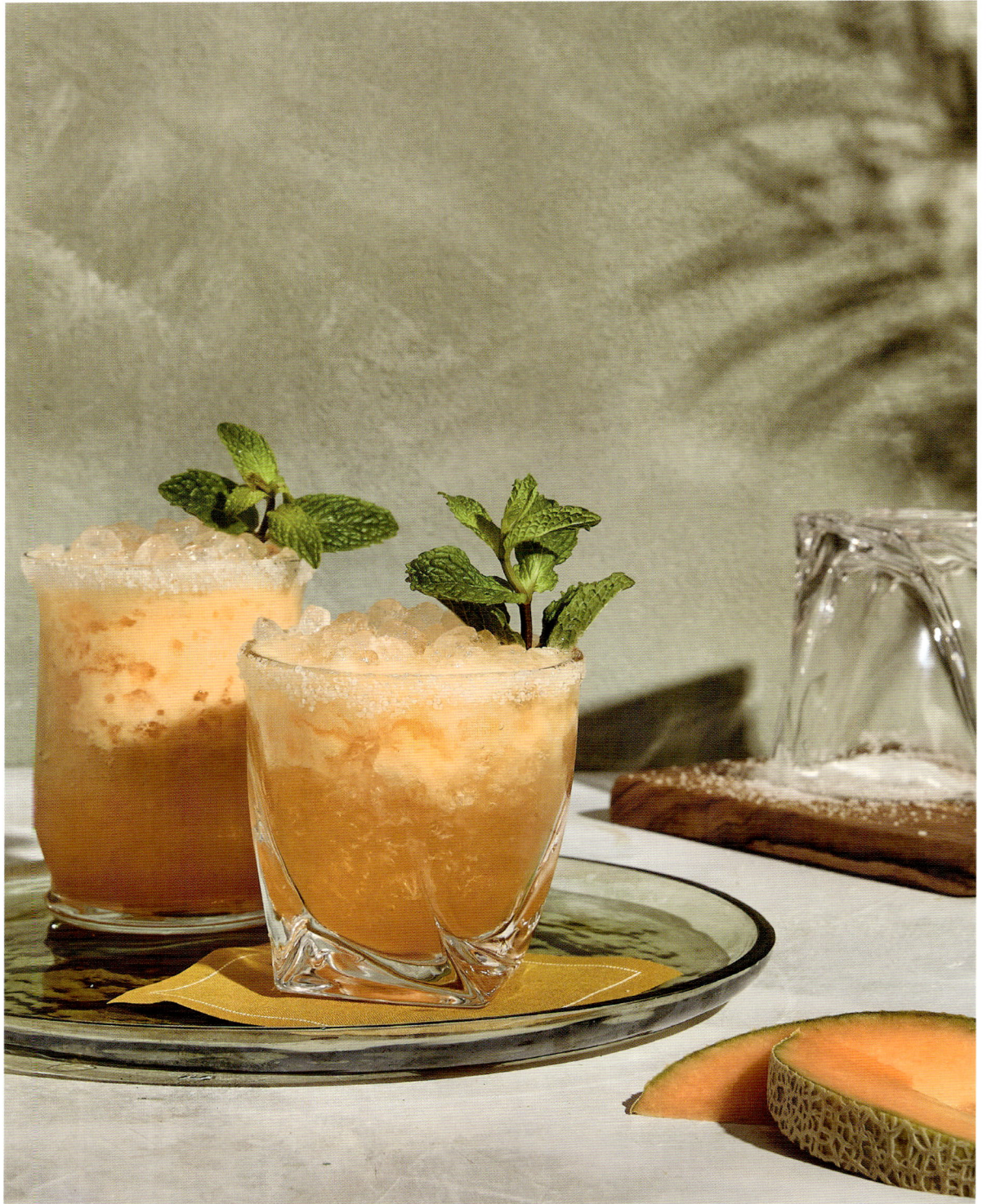

CHARMING *Charly*

SERVES 1

1 cup cubed cantaloupe (7 to 8 chunks)

⅓ cup water (optional)

3 to 5 mint leaves

2 teaspoons agave syrup

Pinch of salt

Ice cubes

⅓ cup club soda, chilled

GARNISH

Agave syrup

Salt

1. To garnish the rim of your glass, place some agave syrup on a small plate. Place some salt on another small plate. Dip the rim of a lowball glass into the agave, then into the salt.

2. Place the cantaloupe, water (if using), mint, 2 teaspoons agave, and pinch of salt in a blender. Blend until smooth.

3. Fill the glass with ice, then strain the cantaloupe mixture into the glass.

4. Top with club soda and enjoy.

Of course I had to name a drink after my golden retriever, Charly. This drink is as fun, playful, and full of energy as the pup it's named after. The juicy cantaloupe paired with the salty rim is just like a great dog: always a crowd-pleaser. This drink is sure to win hearts, just like Charly does!

FIVE WAYS TO
Show Yourself Self-Care

Make yourself a fun mocktail to treat yourself. Put a robe on after dinner and binge your favorite show with a mocktail in hand. Sounds like the ideal night to me!

Enjoy a morning ritual. Start your day with a 10 minute routine just for you, whether it's journaling, putting on those eye patches, going on a quick walk, or having your coffee without distractions.

Plan digital detox time. Pick one hour per day or one weekend morning to unplug. Let your mind rest without scrolling.

Try a new hobby. Painting, pottery, floral arranging, candle making, and bracelet making are fun options!

Do something just for you. Enjoy a skincare mask in bed, go get a mani/pedi, or have a solo coffee date. Habit stacking is my favorite.

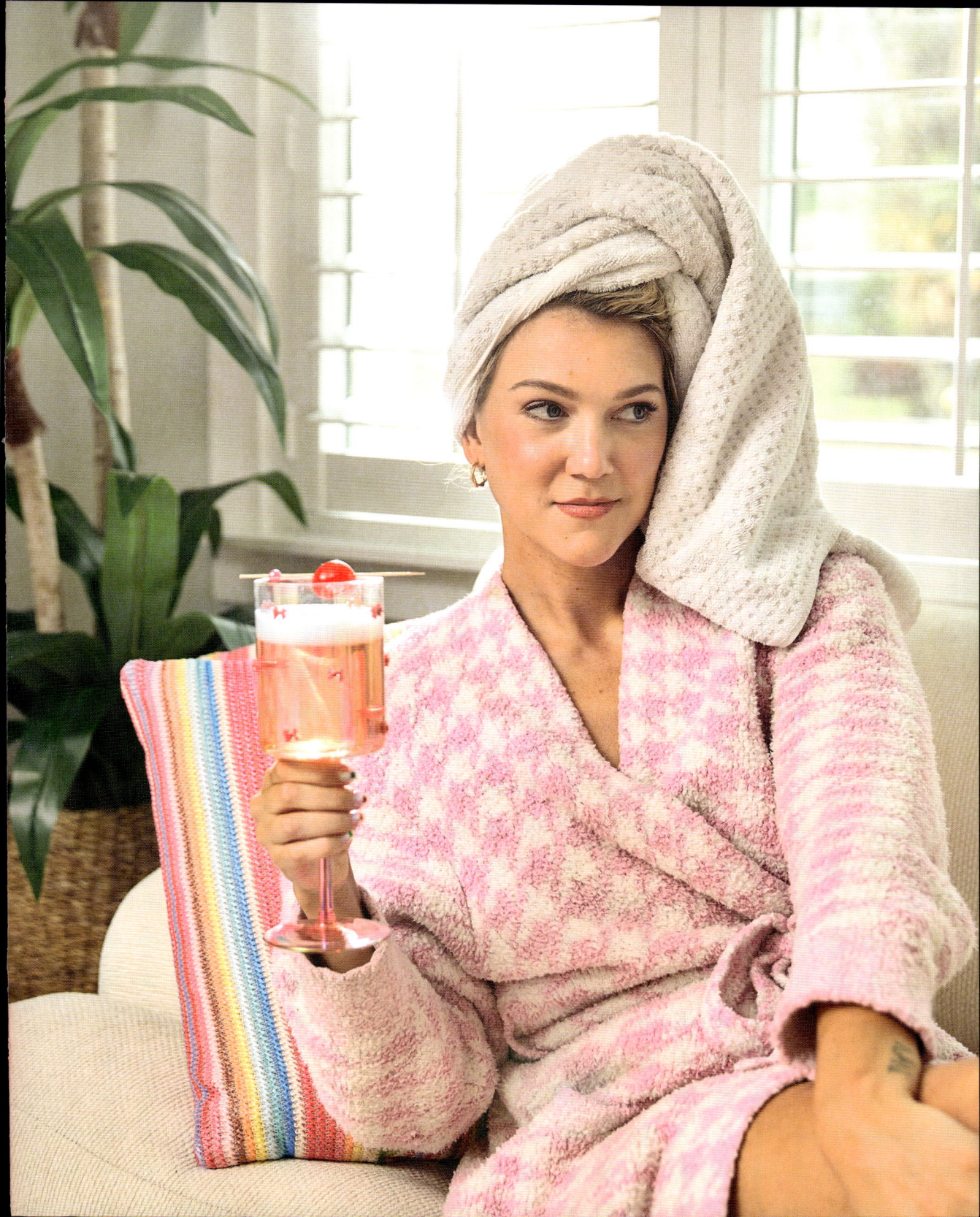

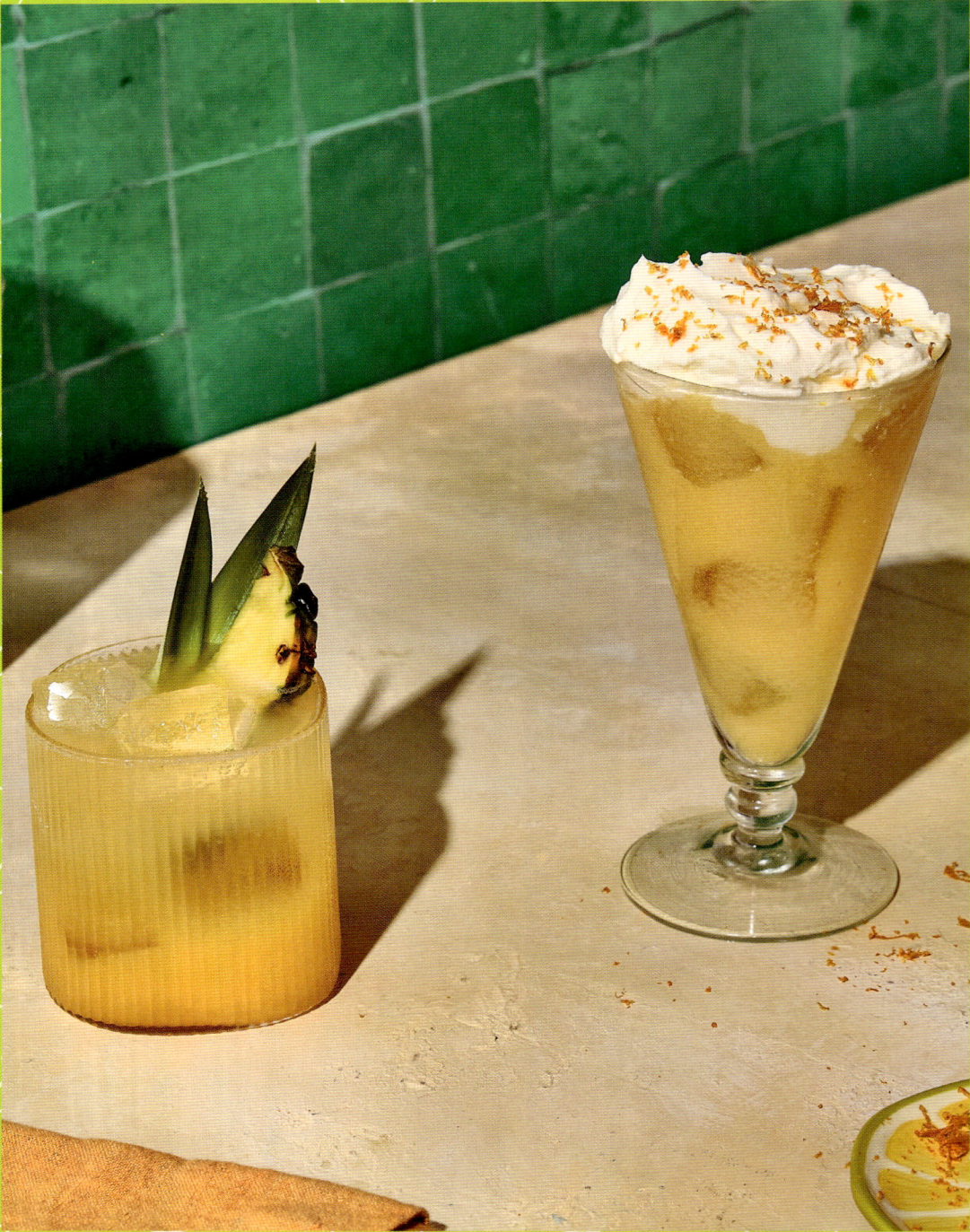

CHAPTER FOUR

R&R

*A*re you stressed and need some rest and relaxation? These mocktails will help you recharge, transporting you to a beach where the only thing that can bring you down is the number of mocktails you can have before it's socially acceptable to take a nap.

VITAMIN *Sea*

SERVES 1

¼ cup blood orange juice

Juice of 1 lime

1 tablespoon agave syrup

4 basil leaves

Ice cubes

⅓ cup unflavored kombucha

GARNISH

1 blood orange slice

Basil leaves

1. Add the blood orange juice, lime juice, agave, and basil to a shaker. Muddle, using a muddler or the back of a wooden spoon, to release the basil aroma, 4 to 5 twists.

2. Add a handful of ice and shake until the outside is frosted and cold, about 5 seconds.

3. Fill a lowball glass with ice. Strain the juice mixture into the glass, then top with kombucha.

4. Garnish with a blood orange slice and basil leaves.

Vitamin Sea is the perfect blend of refreshing and revitalizing, just like a day by the ocean. Packed with flavor, this drink will (not to be dramatic) refresh your soul—no sunscreen required.

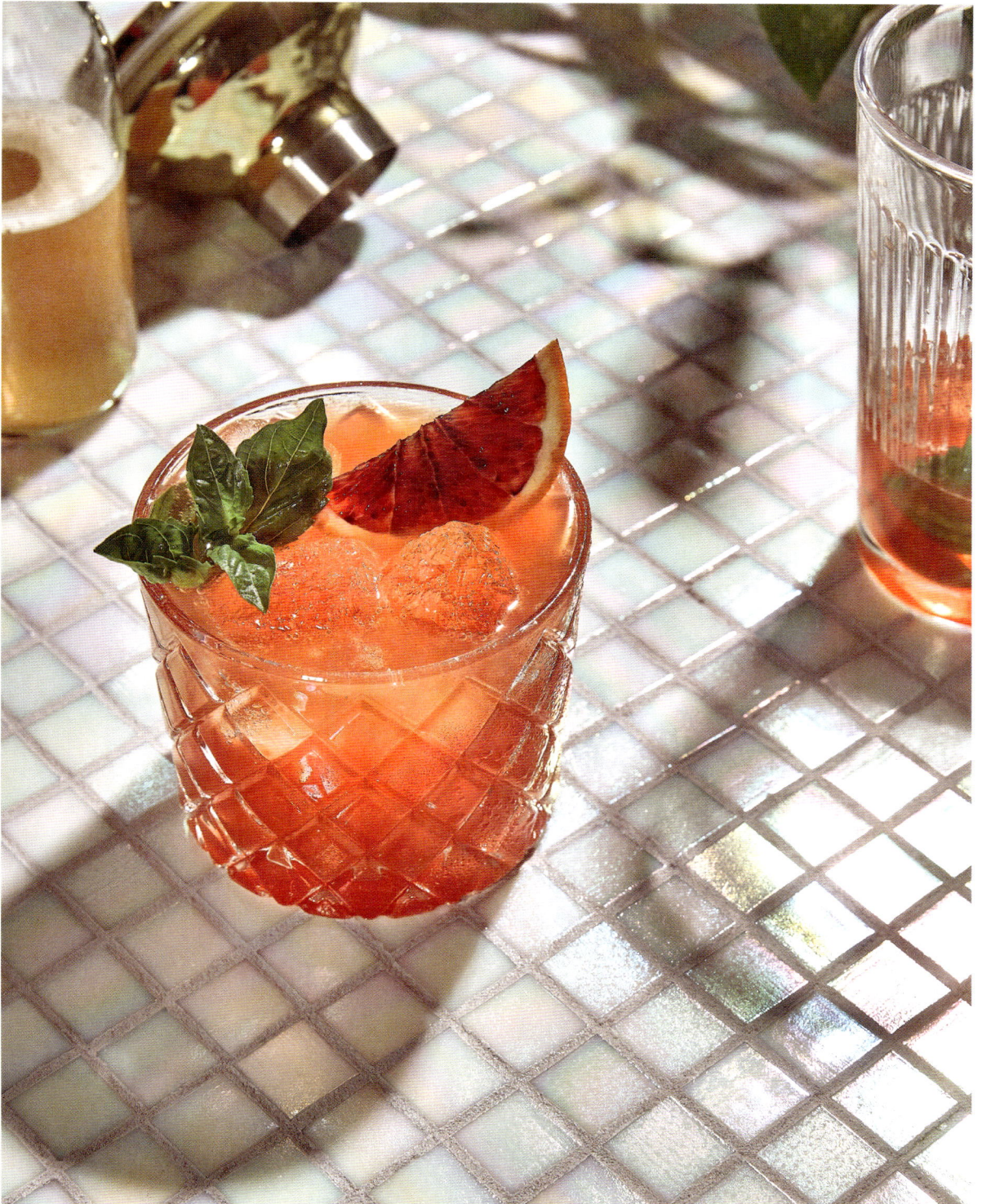

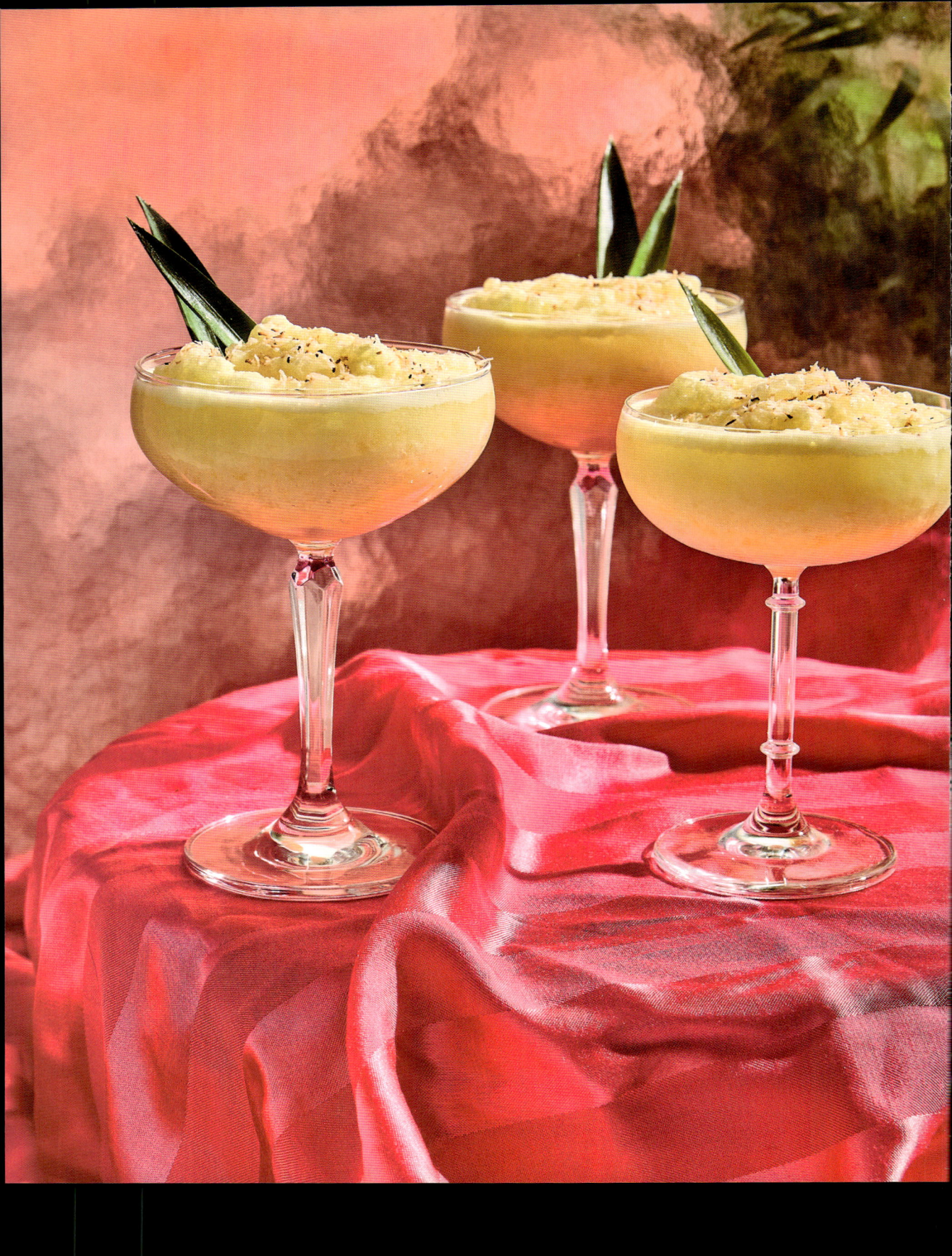

COCONUT *Cooler*

SERVES 1

½ cup pineapple juice

⅓ cup coconut milk

Juice of 1 lime

Ice cubes

⅓ cup coconut sparkling water

GARNISH

1 teaspoon honey

Shredded coconut

1. To garnish the rim of your glass, place the honey on a small plate. Place the coconut on another small plate. Roll the rim of the glass in the honey, then dip it in the coconut to coat. Set aside.

2. Pour the pineapple juice, coconut milk, and lime juice into shaker. Add a handful of ice and shake until the outside of the shaker is frosty, about 5 seconds.

3. Fill the glass with ice, then strain the juice mixture into the glass.

4. Pour the sparkling water on top. Stir and enjoy.

FROZEN COCONUT COOLER

Turn this into a frozen drink by pouring the pineapple juice, coconut milk, and lime juice into a blender. Add 1 cup of ice and blend until smooth. Pour into a glass and top with sparkling water.

I've been a piña colada girl for as long as I can remember, but sometimes I crave the taste without the "frozen" aspect. That's where the Coconut Cooler comes in; it's a smooth and refreshing twist on the classic that leaves you with a little island-inspired bliss.

SWEET & *Strong*

SERVES 1

Ice cubes

1 cup sweet tea

⅓ cup light ginger beer
(I like Fever-Tree)

1 tablespoon apple cider
vinegar

Lemon slices, for garnish

1. Fill a tall glass with ice.

2. Pour the tea, ginger beer, and apple cider vinegar into the glass.

3. Garnish with lemon slices, stir, and enjoy!

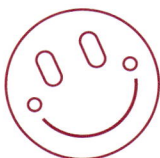

Who says you have to choose between being sweet or being strong? This bold yet refreshing drink brings the smooth, comforting taste of sweet tea together with the fiery kick of ginger beer. This drink proves that strength and sweetness are a winning combo. So go ahead and embrace your whole self—because you, my friend, are both!

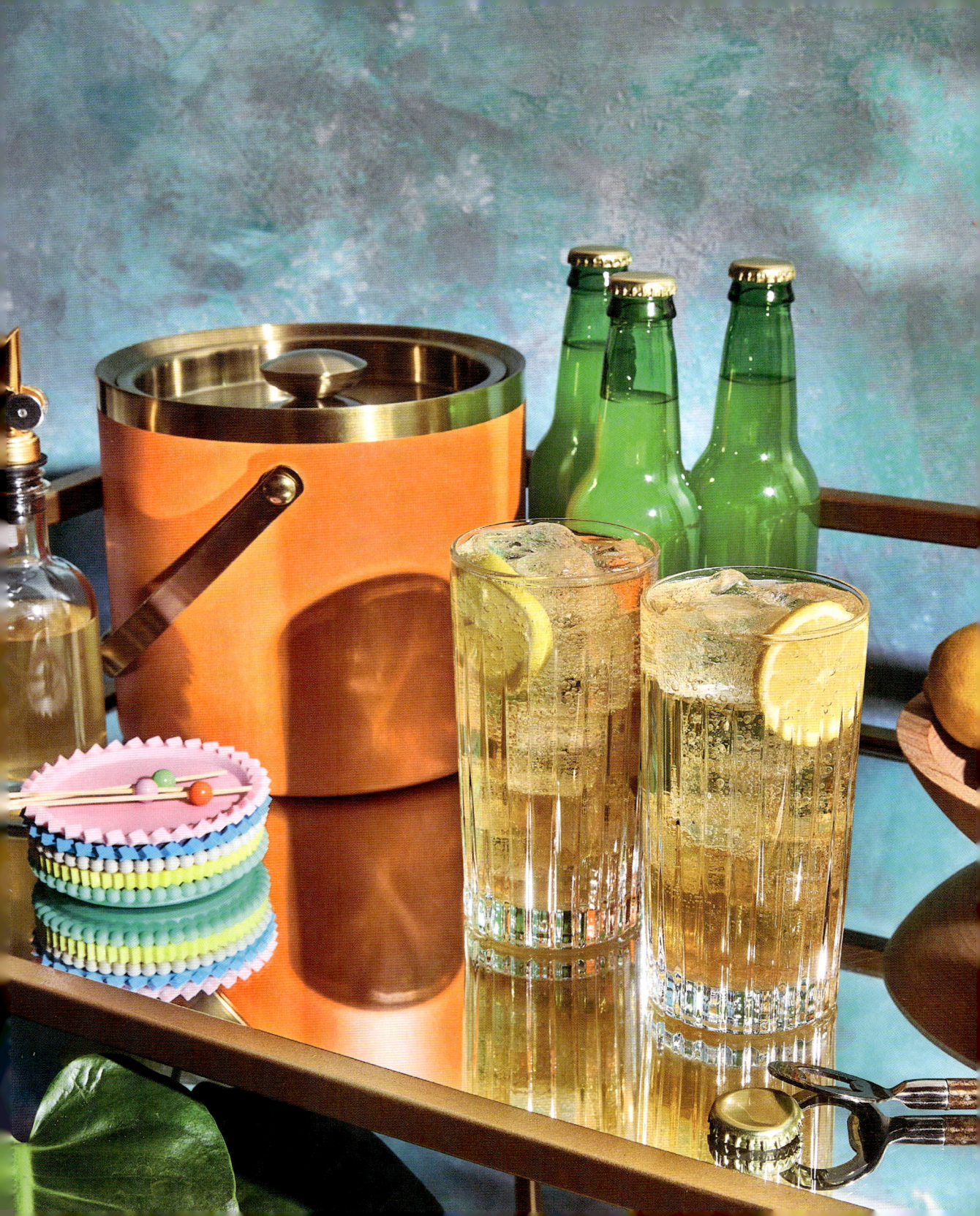

CABANA *Crush*

SERVES 1

¾ cup orange juice

¼ cup coconut milk

1 teaspoon agave syrup

½ teaspoon vanilla extract

Ice cubes

½ cup coconut water or unflavored seltzer

Coconut whipped cream (optional; I like Trader Joe's)

Orange zest (optional)

1. Add the orange juice, coconut milk, agave, and vanilla to a shaker with a handful of ice.

2. Shake until the outside of the shaker is frosty, about 5 seconds.

3. Fill a tall glass with ice and strain in the orange juice mixture.

4. Top with coconut water or seltzer, and add coconut whipped cream and orange zest on top (if using).

This dreamy orange creamsicle mocktail brings all the feel-good vibes in a single sip. Bright, juicy orange meets smooth, creamy vanilla for a nostalgic yet elevated twist on a classic. Creamsicles used to be my jam when I was a kid, and the berry ones weren't so bad either.

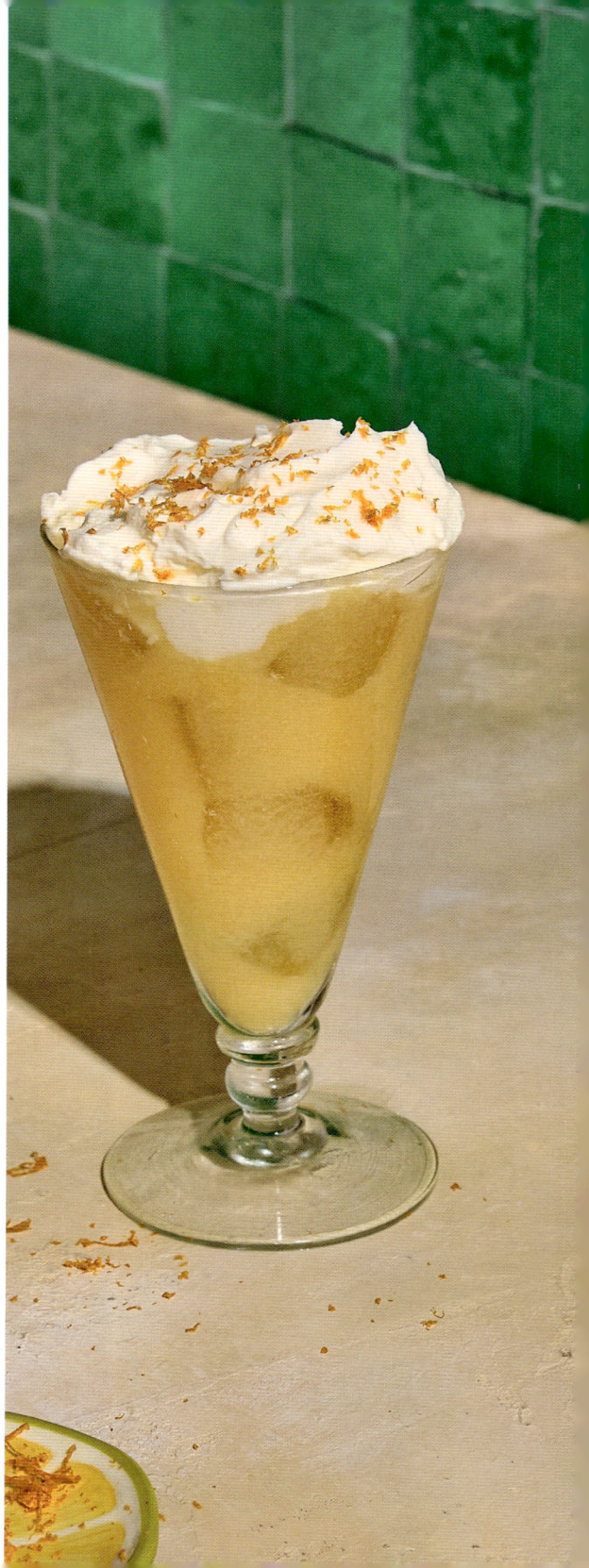

LIQUID
Sunshine

SERVES 1

¼ cup orange juice

¼ cup pineapple juice

Juice of ½ lemon

Ice cubes

¼ cup ginger ale

1. Add the orange juice, pineapple juice, lemon juice, and a handful of ice to a shaker. Shake until the outside of the shaker is frosty, about 5 seconds.

2. Fill a lowball glass with ice. Pour in the juice mixture.

3. Top with ginger ale and enjoy.

I'll never forget the cab driver in The Bahamas who called the rain "liquid sunshine." His positive outlook—finding joy even in a rainstorm—stuck with me. This bright and refreshing mocktail is a little taste of sunshine, no matter the forecast. Cheers to brighter days and little moments of joy with the ones you love!

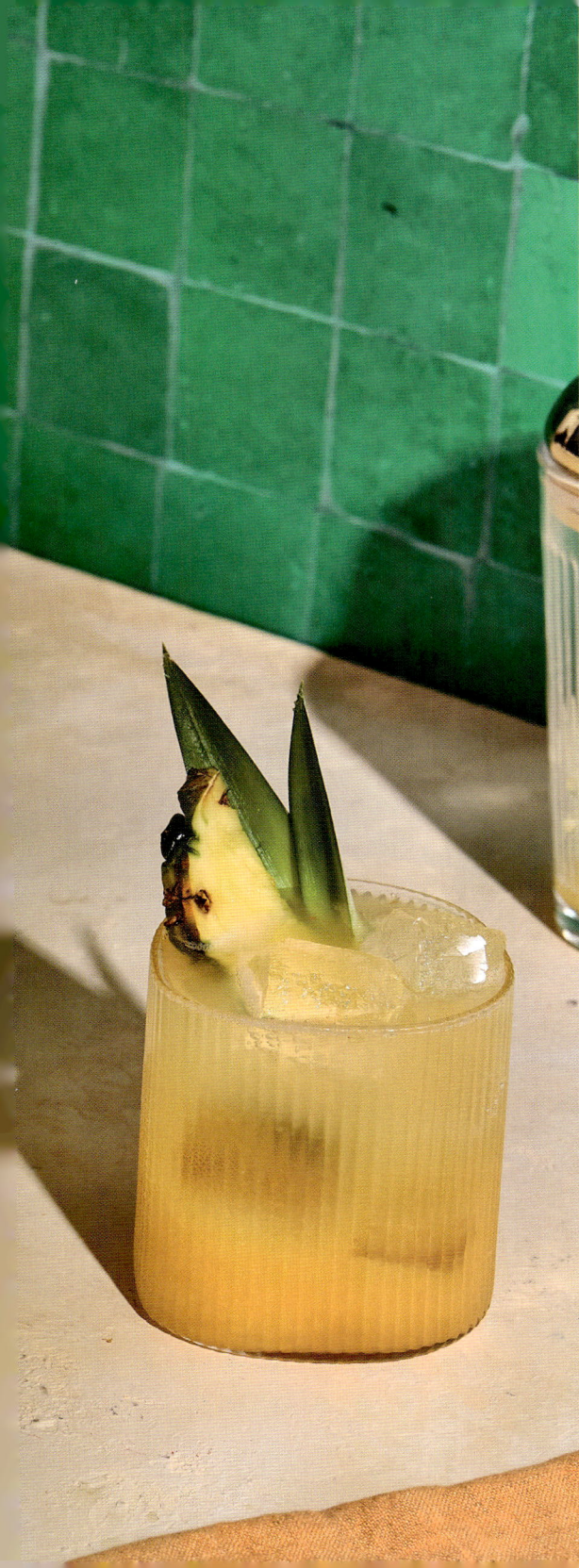

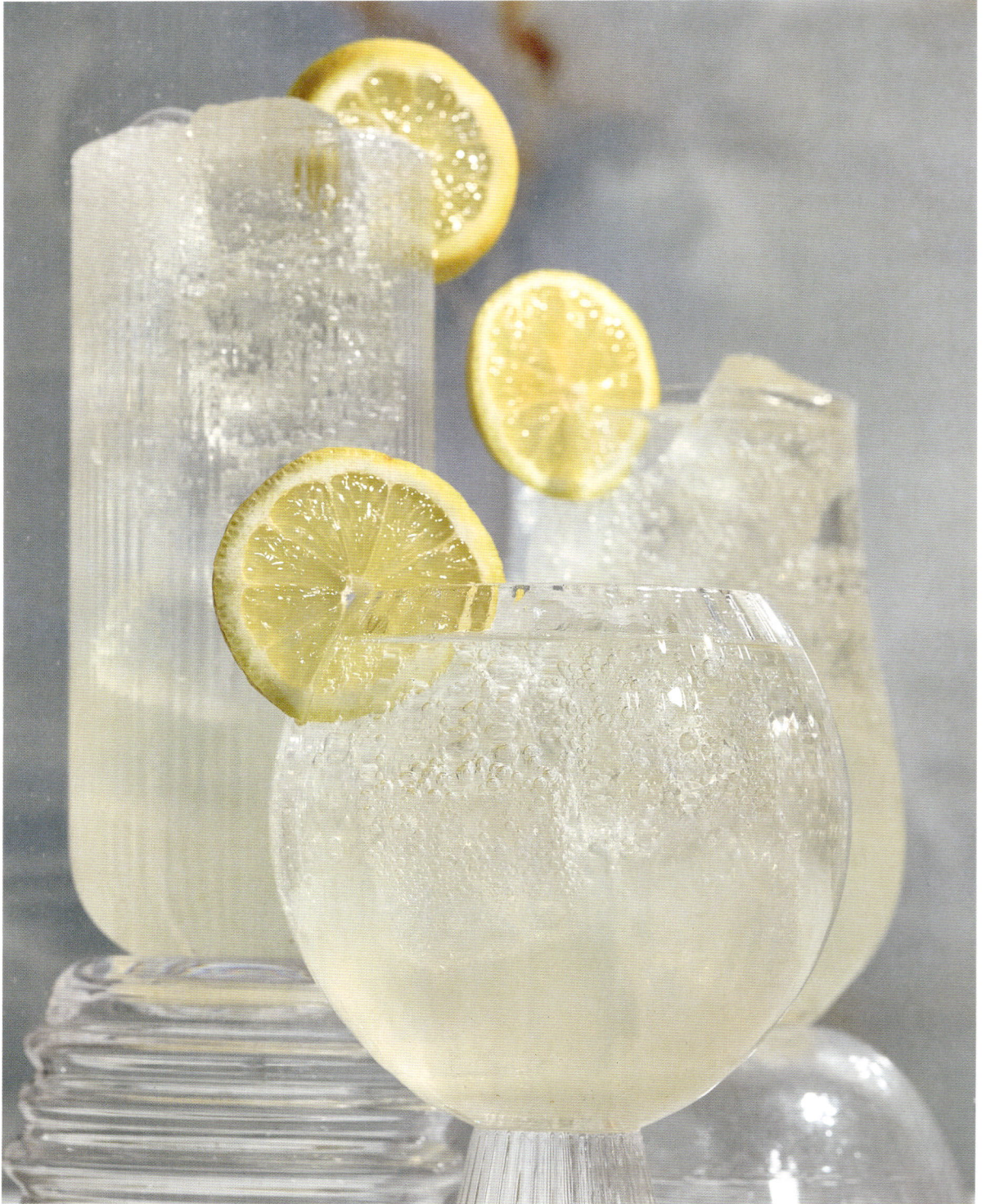

NATURE'S *Lemonade*

SERVES 1

¾ cup coconut water

Juice of 2 lemons

8 mint leaves

Ice cubes

½ cup club soda

GARNISH

1 mint sprig

1 lemon round

1. Add the coconut water, lemon juice, and mint leaves to a shaker.

2. Muddle the mint leaves with a muddler or the back of a wooden spoon by pressing down and rotating until aromatic, 3 to 5 twists.

3. Add a handful of ice, then shake until the outside of the shaker is frosty, about 5 seconds.

4. Fill a highball glass with ice. Strain the mixture into the glass, then top with club soda.

5. Garnish with a mint sprig and a lemon round.

I have a feeling this drink will become a go-to, because who doesn't love lemonade with added hydration? The coconut water adds natural sweetness and electrolytes, making this a refreshing and nourishing sip. I sometimes add a pinch of mineral salt to enhance hydration.

FROZEN PEACH MANGO MARGARITA

ISLAND
Time

SERVES 1

½ cup frozen peach slices

½ cup frozen mango chunks

¾ cup coconut water

Juice of 1 lime

1 teaspoon agave syrup

GARNISH

1 lime wedge

Himalayan salt

1. To garnish the rim of your glass, rub a lime wedge around the rim of a margarita glass. Place the salt on a small plate, then dip the rim into the salt. Set aside (see Tip).

2. Place the peaches, mangos, coconut water, lime juice, and agave in a blender. Blend until smooth and thick.

3. Pour the mixture into the glass.

TIP I like to place the glass in the freezer an hour before serving so it's nice and cold.

This drink is a whole mood. When you sip on this, you'll suddenly have no worries, no deadlines—just beachy vibes and sandy toes. Whether you're actually ocean-side or manifesting it from your couch, this is your official pass to sit back, relax, and live in the moment.

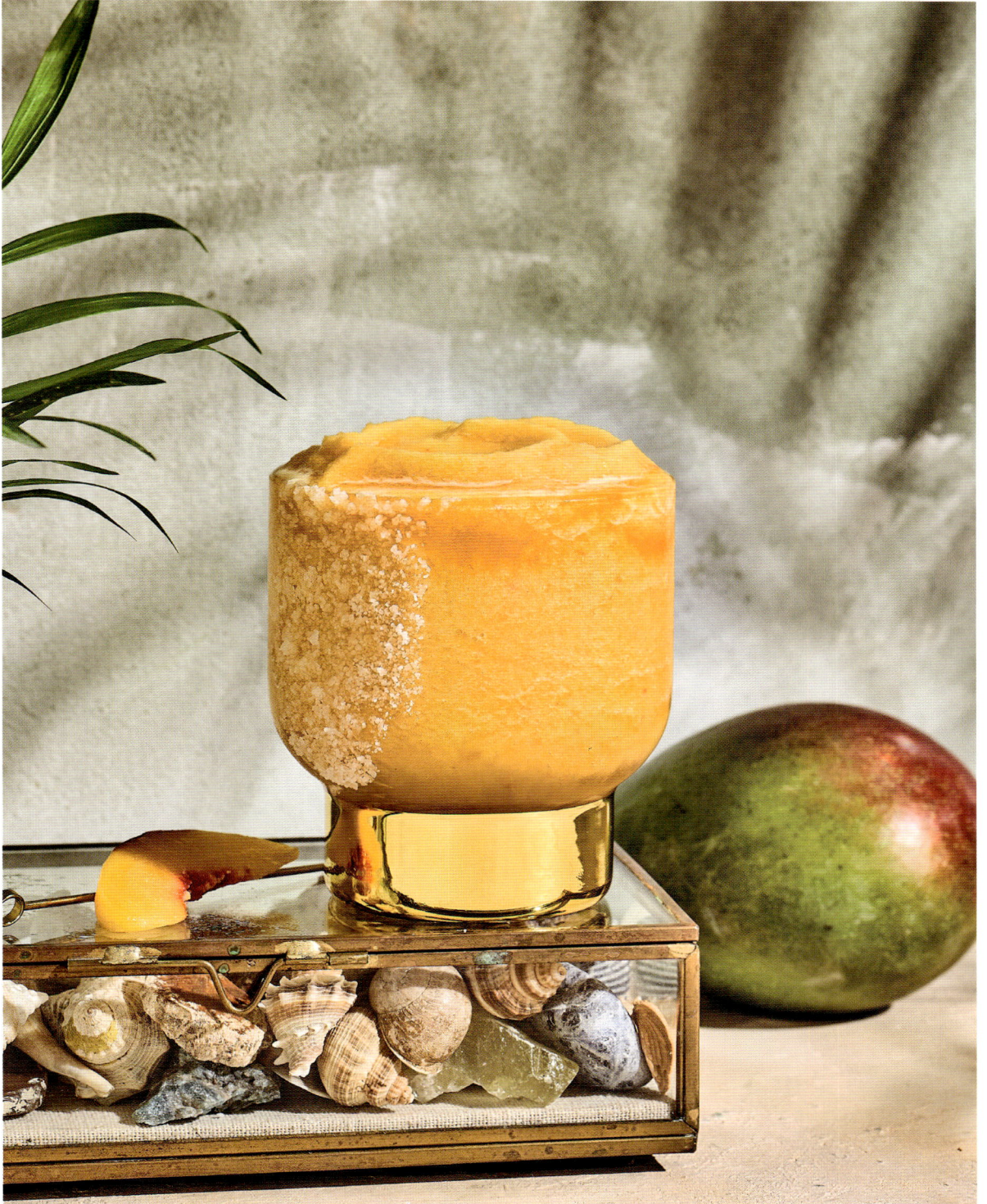

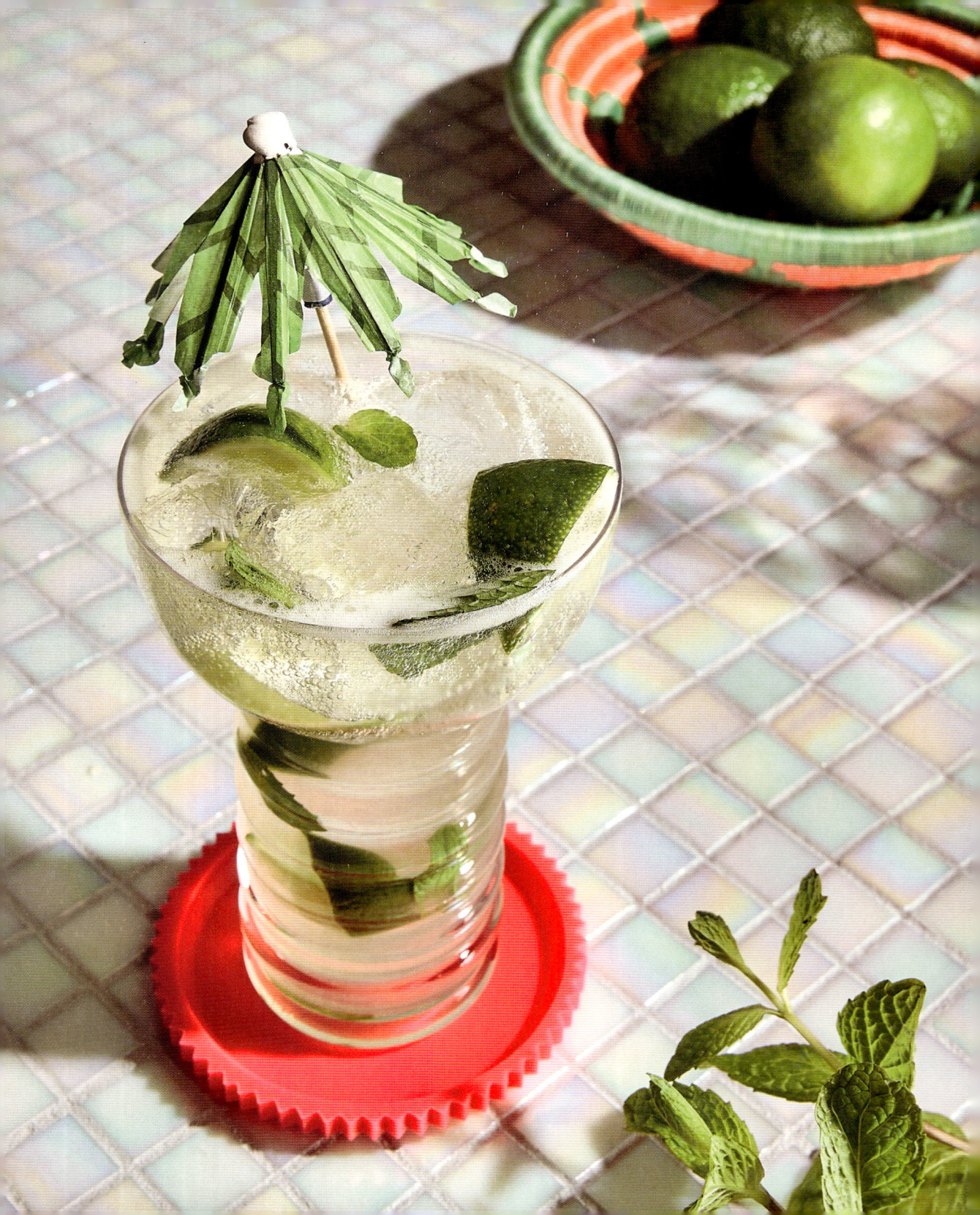

The TIKI TOK

SERVES 1

1 lime, sliced into wedges

10 to 12 mint leaves

1 tablespoon agave syrup

½ cup coconut water

Ice cubes

½ cup lemon-lime sparkling water

1. Squeeze the juice from the lime wedges into a shaker, then drop the wedges in.

2. Add the mint leaves and agave and muddle with a muddler or the back of a wooden spoon by gently pressing down and rotating to release the mint aroma, 3 to 5 times. (I avoid muddling too much, since I like my mint leaves to stay intact.)

3. Add the coconut water and a handful of ice. Shake until the outside of the shaker is frosty, about 5 seconds. Pour the entire mixture, including the ice, into a tall glass.

4. Add another handful of ice and top with the sparkling water. Stir and enjoy.

This "nojito," if you will, is my go-to when I am on vacation or need a quick, refreshing mocktail that will take about 5 minutes. The best one I ever had was in The Bahamas. I had the bartender make me another (I mean, it's a mocktail, so drink up!) just so I could see his technique. So we can say this was inspired by our guy Bruno, the bartender near the wave pool at Atlantis.

THE 561

SERVES 1

1 cup coconut water

Juice of ½ lemon

Juice of ½ lime

1 teaspoon agave syrup

1 teaspoon blue spirulina

Ice cubes

1. Add the coconut water, lemon juice, lime juice, agave, and spirulina to a highball glass.

2. Use a frother to mix the spirulina into the liquids. (If you don't have a frother, you can use a blender or immersion blender.)

3. Fill the glass with ice. Stir and enjoy!

This drink is named after Palm Beach County, where I grew up. I'm a Florida gal! I moved to NYC at the age of 18 and thought I would never move back—but I was wrong. Whether it be my sunshiny personality, my love of slow living, my sweaty lifestyle, or my obsession with the ocean, I love calling Florida my home. My favorite thing to do is swim in the beautiful blue water, so I just had to make a drink that is a similar color using spirulina, a kind of blue-green algae. Aside from making the drink blue, spirulina has so many antioxidant properties, and its sweet flavor pairs perfectly with the citrus to create a super-hydrating mocktail.

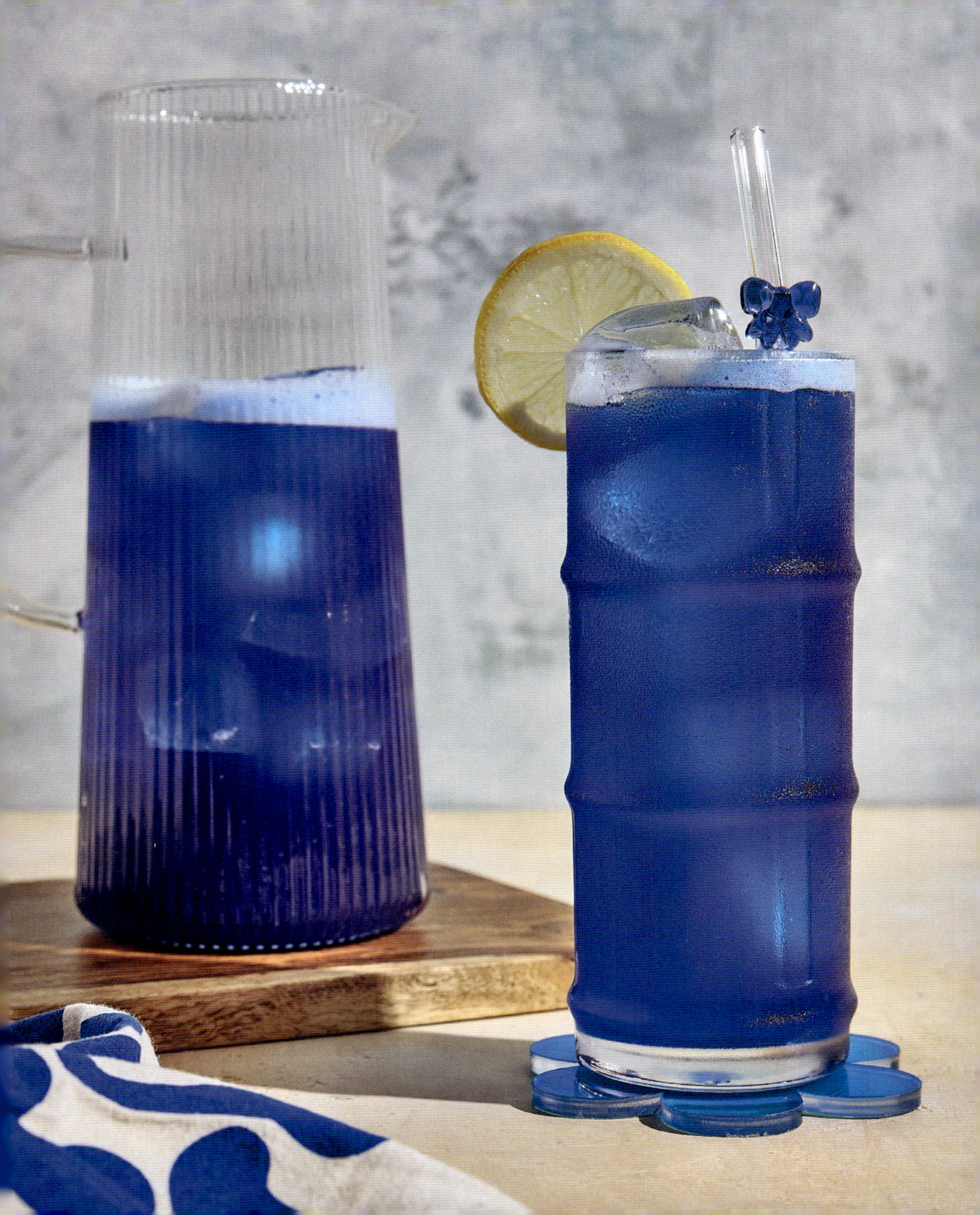

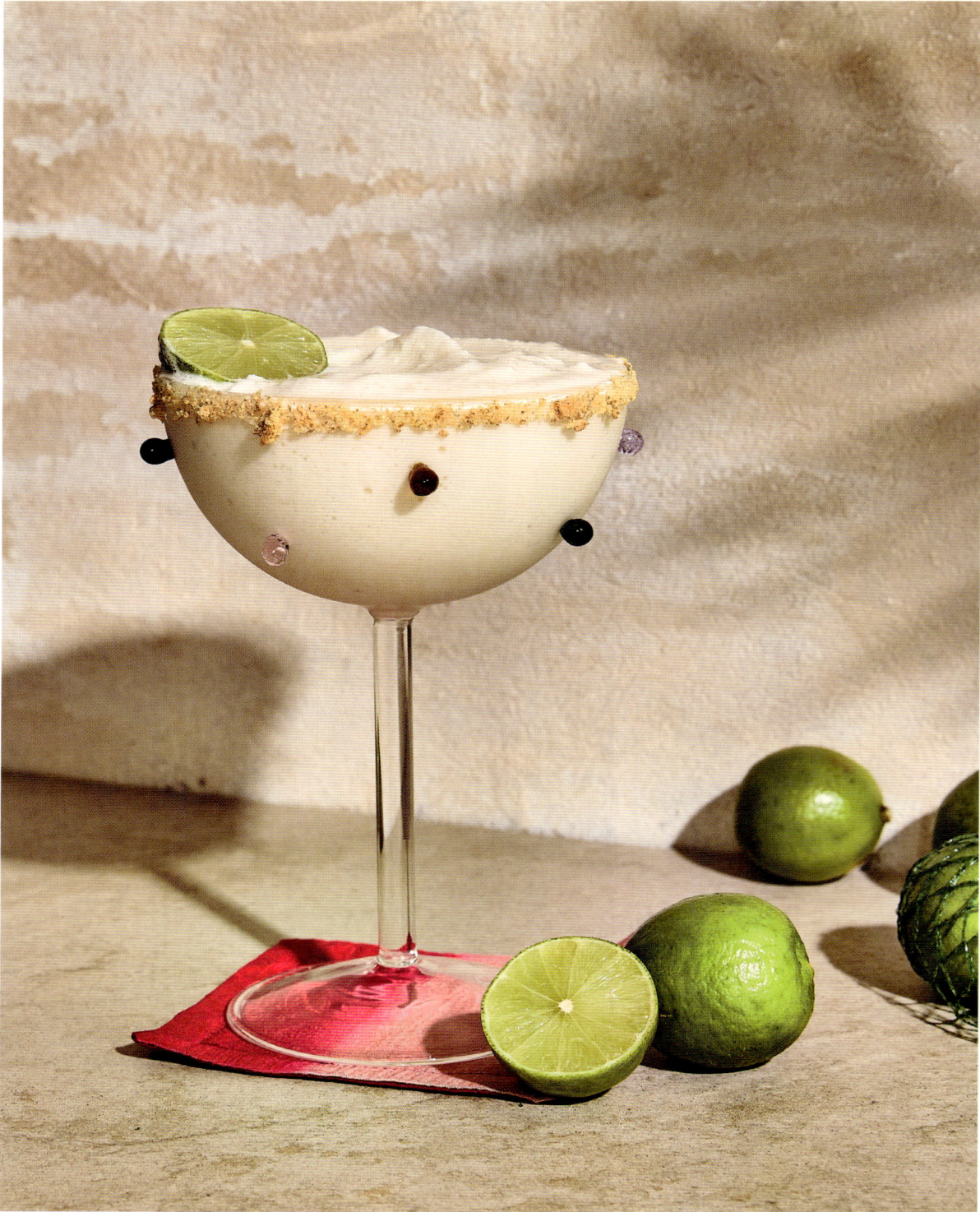

SLICE OF THE *Tropics*

SERVES 1

Juice of 2 limes

⅓ cup cream of coconut
(I use Goya)

1 teaspoon vanilla extract

1 cup ice cubes

GARNISH

1 lime wedge, for the rim
(optional)

1 tablespoon crushed
graham crackers, for the
rim (optional)

1 lime round

1. To garnish the rim of your glass, if desired, rub the lime wedge around the edge of a coupe glass. Place the graham crackers onto a plate and dip the rim into the crackers. Set aside.

2. Place the lime juice, cream of coconut, vanilla, and ice in a blender and blend until smooth and slushy.

3. Pour into the glass and garnish with a lime round.

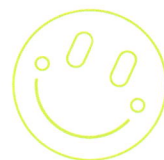

A few years ago, I took a trip down to the Florida Keys with my best friend and we had the best key lime pie daiquiri; I knew I needed to make a mocktail version of it ASAP. I will warn you: This drink has the power to make you crave a daiquiri every second of every day—whether you like key lime pie or not.

TIPS TO GET THE

Best Sleep of Your Life

Get squeaky clean. There is no better way to get ready for bed than taking a warm shower. If you want to switch it up, take a luxurious bubble bath with bubbles, candles, and a calming playlist.

Elevate your evening with a mocktail. Sipping and slaying can now be a part of your bedtime ritual. Treat yourself by indulging in any of the recipes from the Self-Care Sips chapter, starting on page 61.

Get cozy. Just like how putting on a cute workout set makes you feel more motivated to work out, getting in your softest pajamas can help you wind down. Soft is the name of the game.

Swap your phone for a book. Ditch that phone at least an hour before bedtime. Since I made the switch to reading, I've not only had better energy but have bonded with other romance novel lovers.

Set the scene. Two things that completely changed my quality of sleep are blackout curtains and a sound machine. My husband swears by a sleep mask, too.

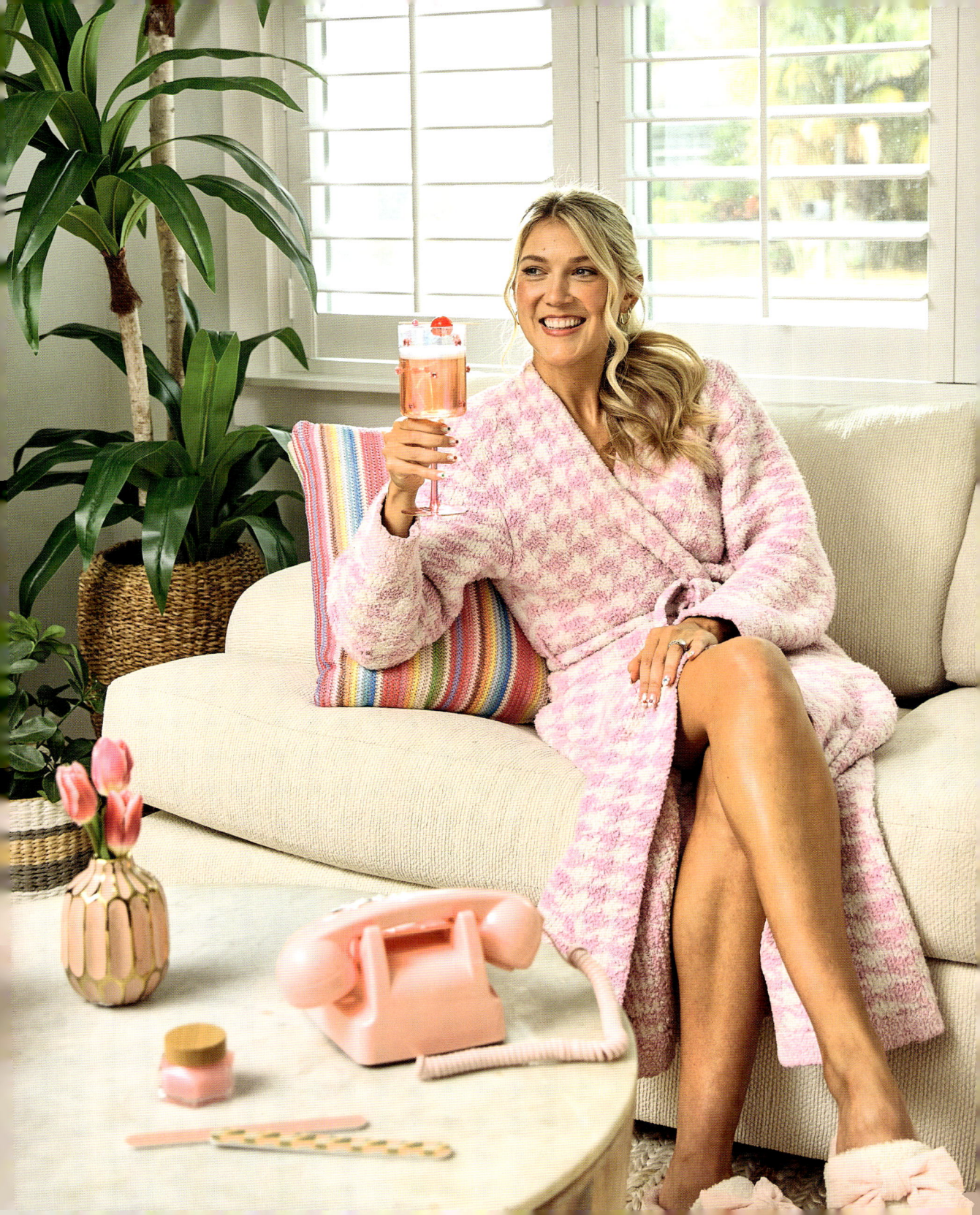

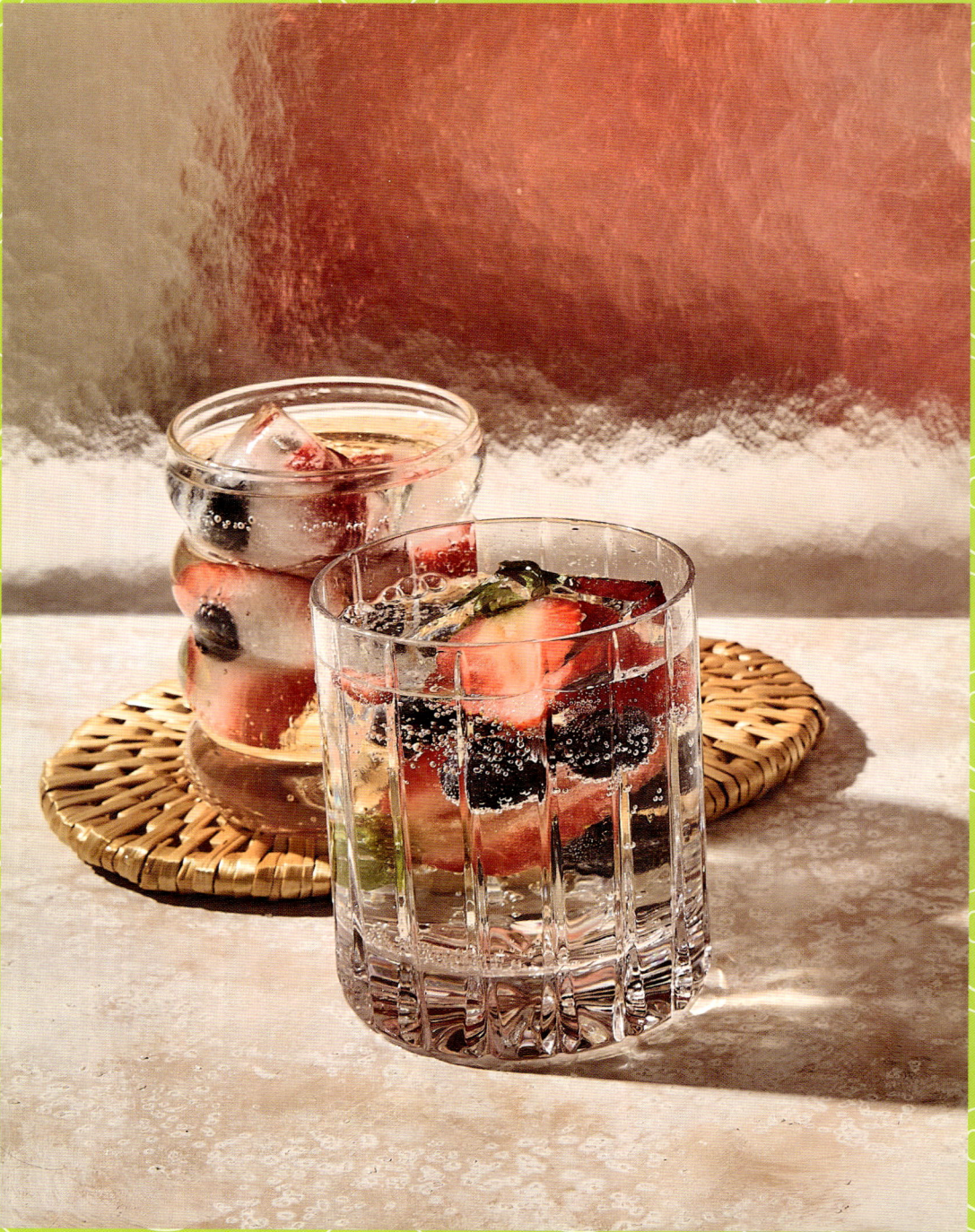

CHAPTER FIVE

SEASONAL
Sips

*D*rinking mocktails for every season and every holiday isn't a want but a *need*. These mocktails are fun and festive, allowing you to stay fully present and enjoy every moment.

APPLE FIZZ

BYOE *Elixir*

SERVES 1

¼ cup apple juice

Juice of ½ lemon

1 tablespoon grenadine

1 egg white

Ice cubes

¼ cup club soda

1 cherry, for garnish

1. Add the apple juice, lemon juice, grenadine, and egg white to a shaker along with a handful of ice.

2. Shake to mix the egg white until foamy, about 30 seconds.

3. Strain the drink into a coupe glass.

4. Top with club soda and garnish with a cherry.

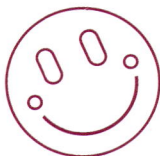

I live by my mantra, BYOE (bring your own energy), and this drink screams just that. The vibrant color, sweet flavor, and frothy egg white foam give off the type of energy that I want to be around. Remember, the energy you bring is everything. With every sip of this BYOE Elixir, you're choosing to be that good energy and spread that good energy. Cheers to that!

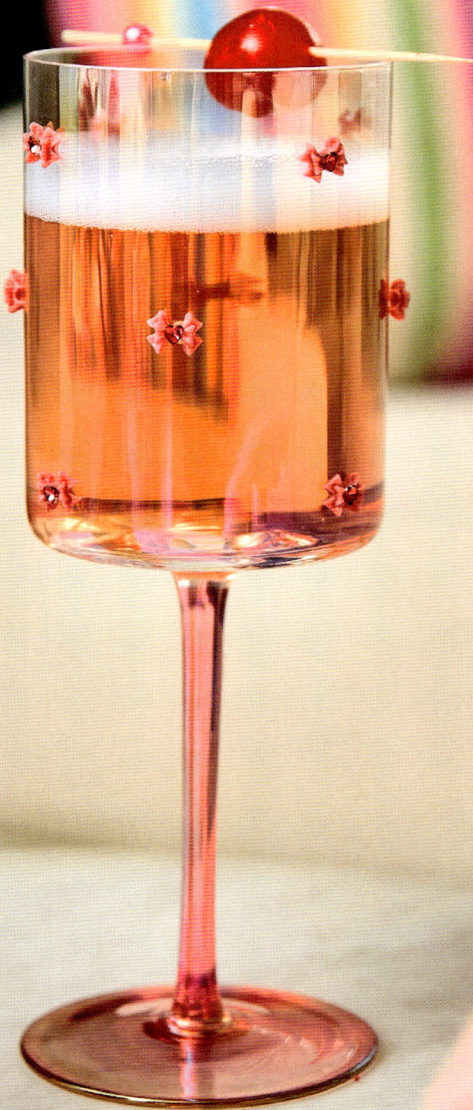

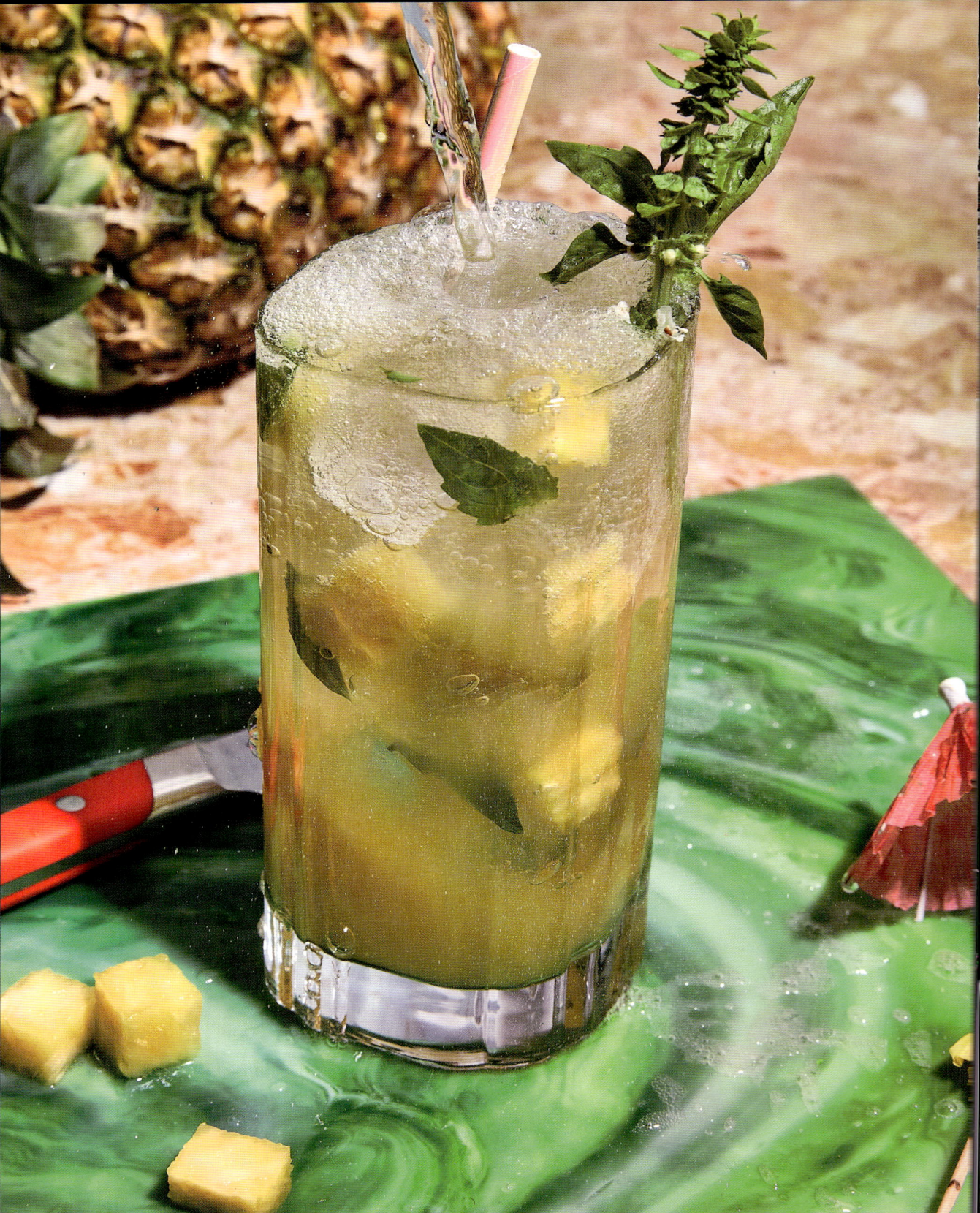

LUCK OF THE *Irish*

SERVES 1

½ cup cubed pineapple

Juice of 1 lemon

2 tablespoons pineapple juice

1½ teaspoons agave syrup

4 basil leaves, chopped

Ice cubes

⅓ cup club soda

GARNISH

1 lime wedge

1 basil sprig

1. Add the pineapple cubes, lemon juice, pineapple juice, agave, and basil to a highball glass.

2. Muddle with a muddler or the back of a wooden spoon until the pineapple cubes are crushed and juicy.

3. Fill the glass with ice, then top with club soda.

4. Garnish with a lime wedge and basil sprig.

I believe luck is when hard work meets opportunity, and this mocktail is the perfect example: The sweet pineapple chunks and fresh basil come together to create something amazing with just the right mix of flavors.

MOM-O-SA

SERVES 1

½ cup store-bought green juice, chilled

¼ cup orange juice

¼ cup pineapple kombucha

1. Pour the green juice and orange juice into a champagne flute

2. Stir and then top with the kombucha.

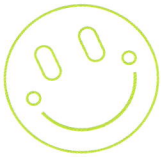

The Mom-O-sa: because taking care of you is just as important as taking care of everyone else. It's a quick, refreshing combination of greens and bubbles, a reminder that even the busiest moms deserve a moment of self-care.

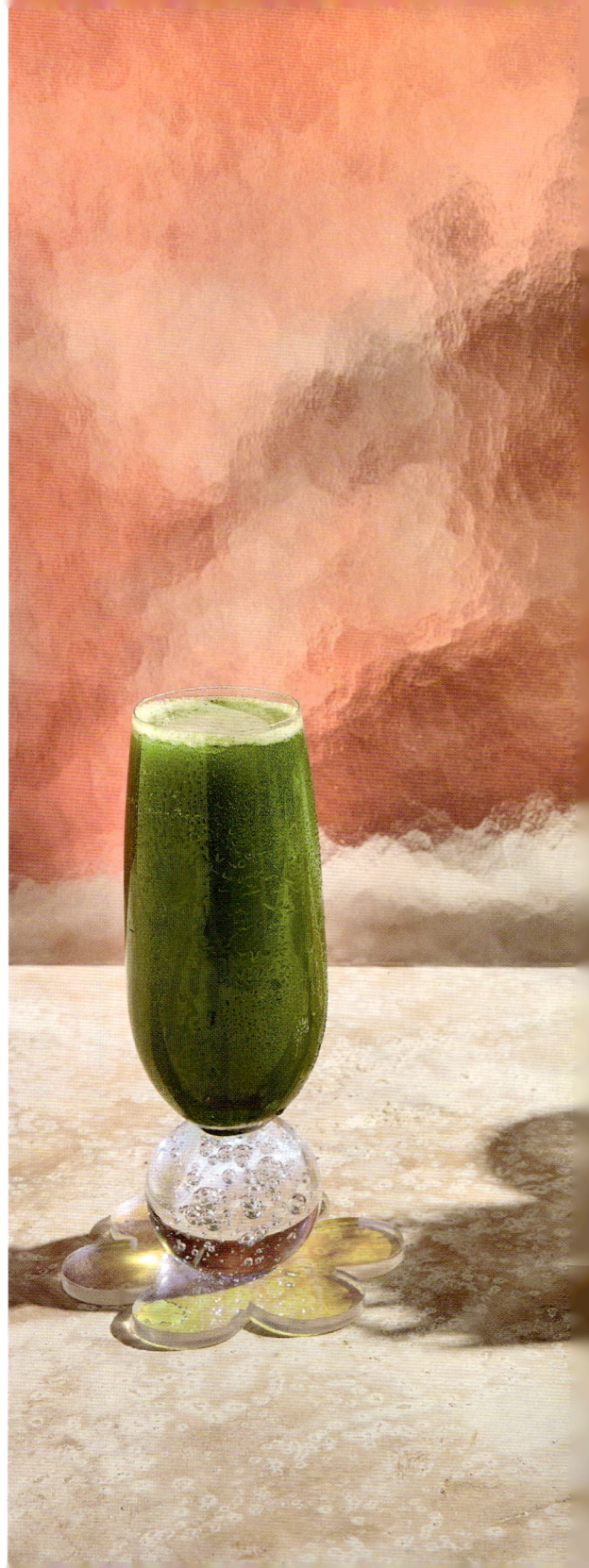

TRIPLE BERRY ICE CUBE HYDRATOR

PARTY IN *the USA*

SERVES 1

Handful of raspberries

Handful of blueberries

2 strawberries, chopped

½ cup coconut water

1 cup lemon-lime soda (I like Olipop Ridge Rush; see Note)

1. Fill an ice cube tray with the raspberries, blueberries, and strawberries, then pour the coconut water on top. This should make about five ice cubes.

2. Place in the freezer until frozen, about 4 hours.

3. Place the ice cubes in a lowball glass and top with the soda.

NOTE You can substitute sparkling water with lemon and lime juice squeezed in for the lemon-lime soda!

The triple berry ice cubes in this recipe turn any drink into a festive fruit celebration, and here, they slowly melt into a lemon-lime base. It's hydration with a pop of color and a whole lot of fun. This drink is perfect for any occasion because it's so simple. It really is the easiest way to bring a party to your cup.

HOCUS POCUS

SERVES 1

6 to 8 concord grapes

¼ cup concord grape juice

Juice of ½ lemon

1 tablespoon agave syrup

1 egg white

Ice cubes

¼ cup club soda

Lemon twist, for garnish

1. Place the grapes in a shaker and muddle with a muddler or the back of a wooden spoon until they release a dark purple juice, about 30 seconds.

2. Add the grape juice, lemon juice, agave, and egg white.

3. Shake for 15 seconds, add a handful of ice, and then shake again for another 15 seconds, until the outside of the shaker is frosty.

4. Strain the mixture into a coupe glass, top with club soda, and garnish with a lemon twist.

I know without a doubt the Sanderson sisters would love this magical mocktail that brings a little fizz and a lot of fun. The bold sweetness of the grapes with the egg white foam makes this the ideal drink to sip on while watching your favorite spooky movie. For me, that would be Hocus Pocus *for about the hundredth time.*

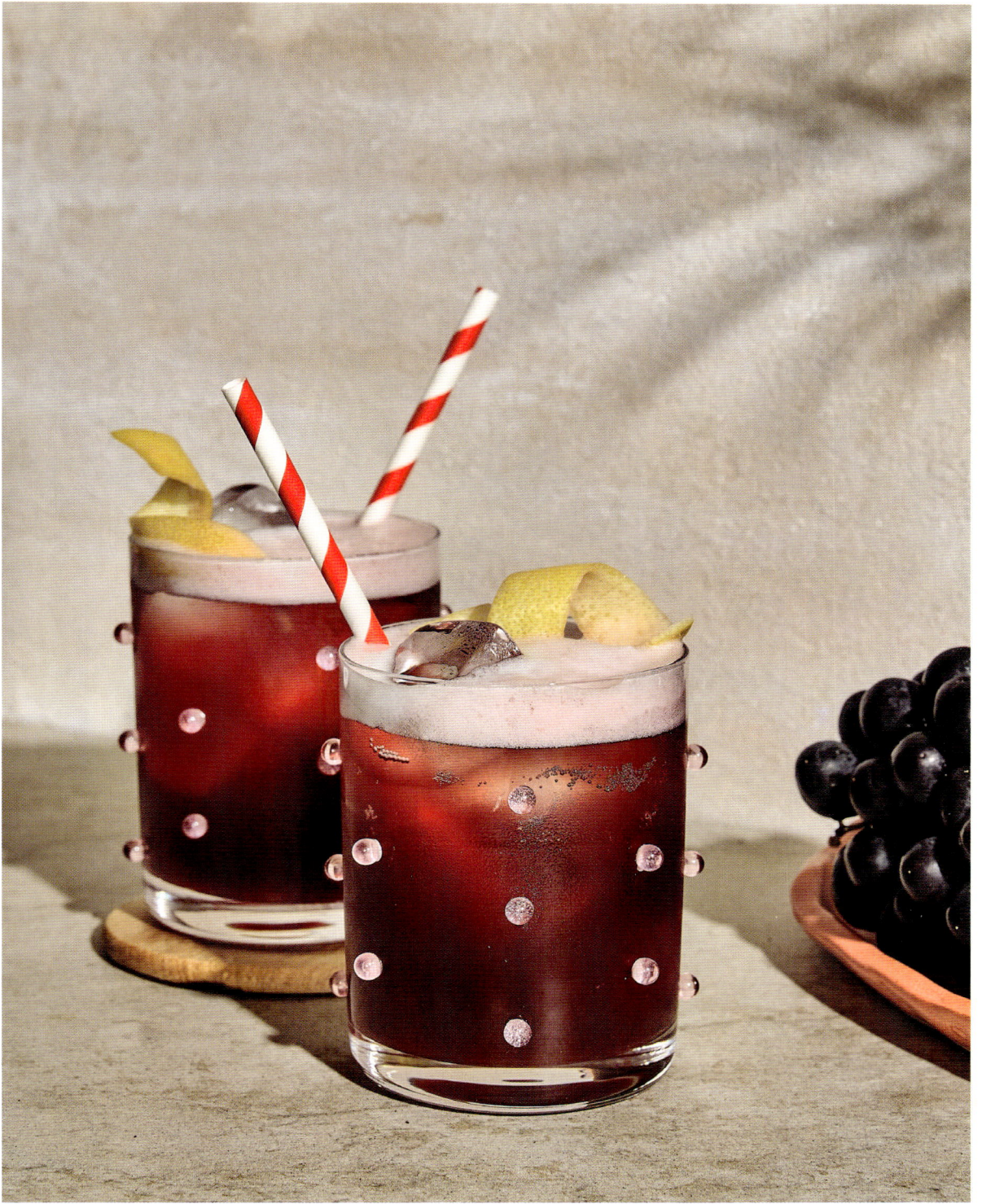

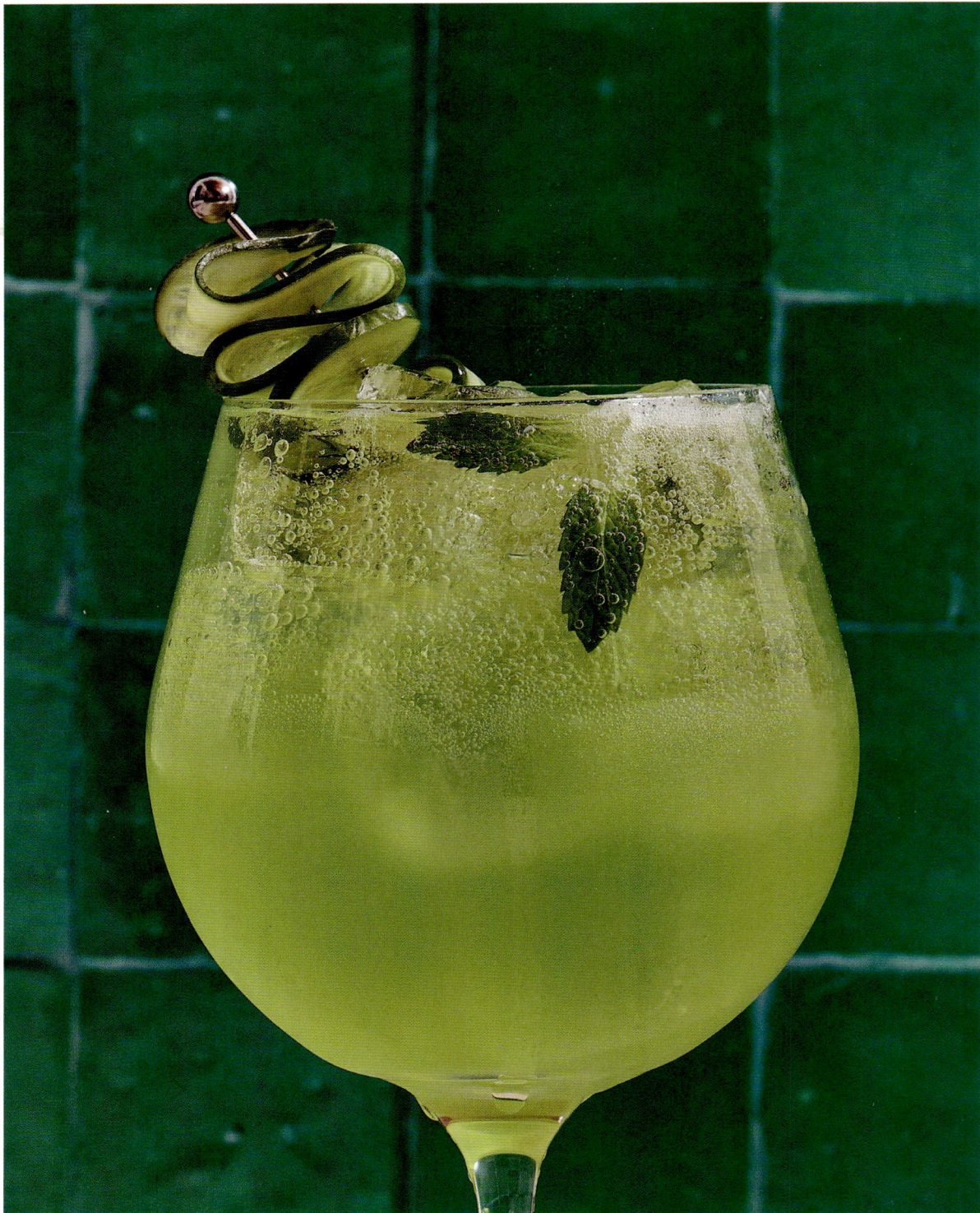

GARDEN *Cooler*

SERVES 1

Juice of 1 lime

5 mint leaves

⅓ cup cucumber juice

3 tablespoons elderflower syrup

Ice cubes

⅓ cup unflavored sparkling water

1. Place the lime juice and mint leaves in a large wineglass. Muddle until the minty aroma is released, 4 to 6 twists.

2. Pour the cucumber juice and elderflower syrup on top.

3. Fill the glass with ice and top with sparkling water.

Garden Cooler is basically the drink version of all those chill garden vibes I've been soaking in lately. I'm not a gardening expert, but I've totally fallen in love with the whole process. This spritz, with its refreshing cucumber and light elderflower flavors, feels like a cool breeze on a sunny day spent outside among the plants. It's the perfect sip that will have you feeling all types of fresh.

PUMPKIN PIE SMOOTHIE

HASHTAG *Basic*

SERVES 1

¾ cup milk of choice

¼ cup vanilla protein powder (optional)

2 tablespoons plain Greek yogurt

1 tablespoon pumpkin puree

1½ teaspoons honey

¼ teaspoon pumpkin pie spice

Handful of ice cubes

1. Add the milk, protein powder (if using), yogurt, pumpkin puree, honey, pumpkin pie spice, and ice cubes to a blender. Blend until the mixture is smooth and the ice is broken down.

2. Pour the smoothie into a tall glass and enjoy!

Listen, I know I start pumpkin spice season too early every year, but I only get to enjoy it for a short period of time, so let me live! This pumpkin pie smoothie is sweet, smooth, and totally Instagrammable, and it's exactly what your taste buds need. So, go ahead and sip your basic-ness with pride! I know I do!

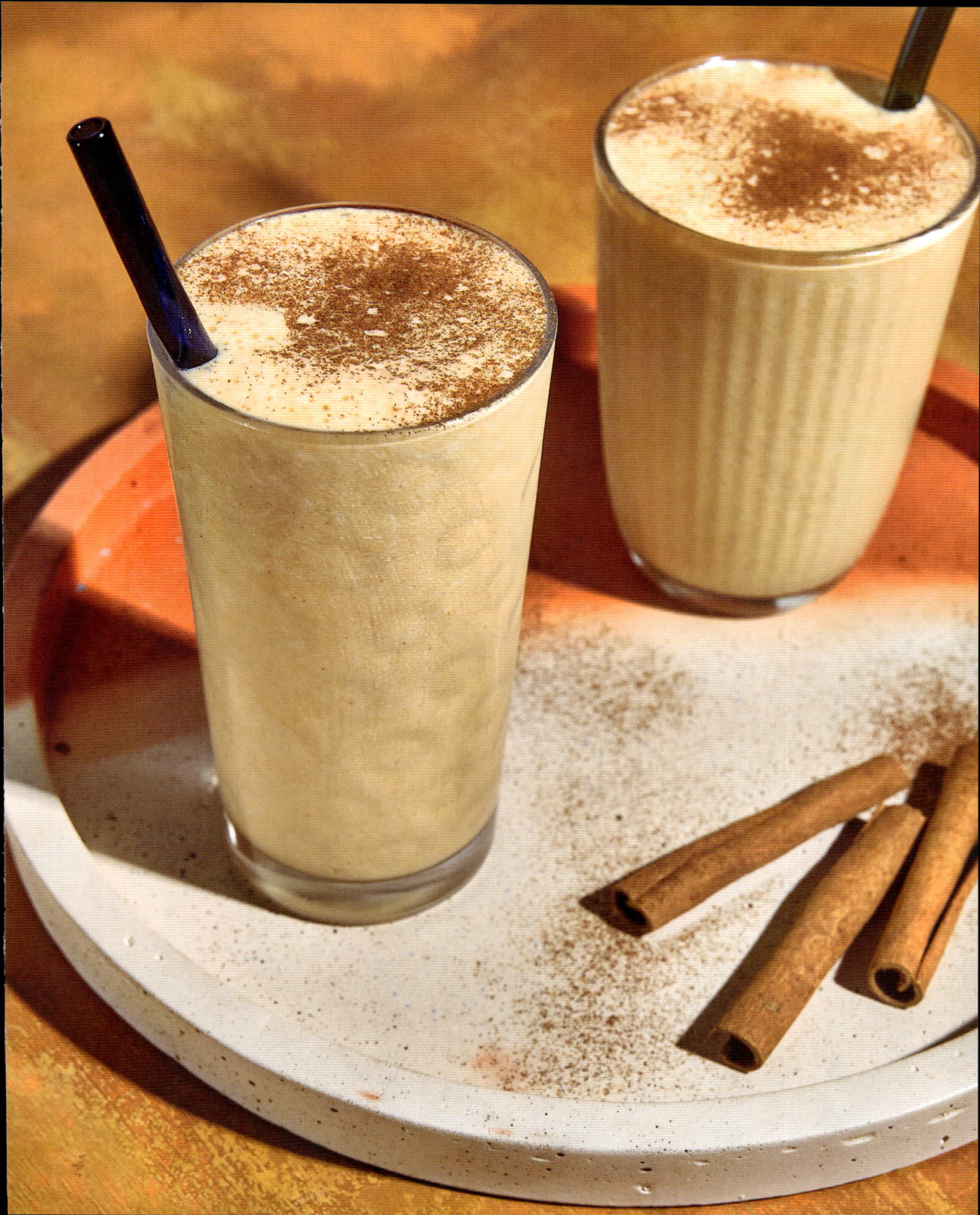

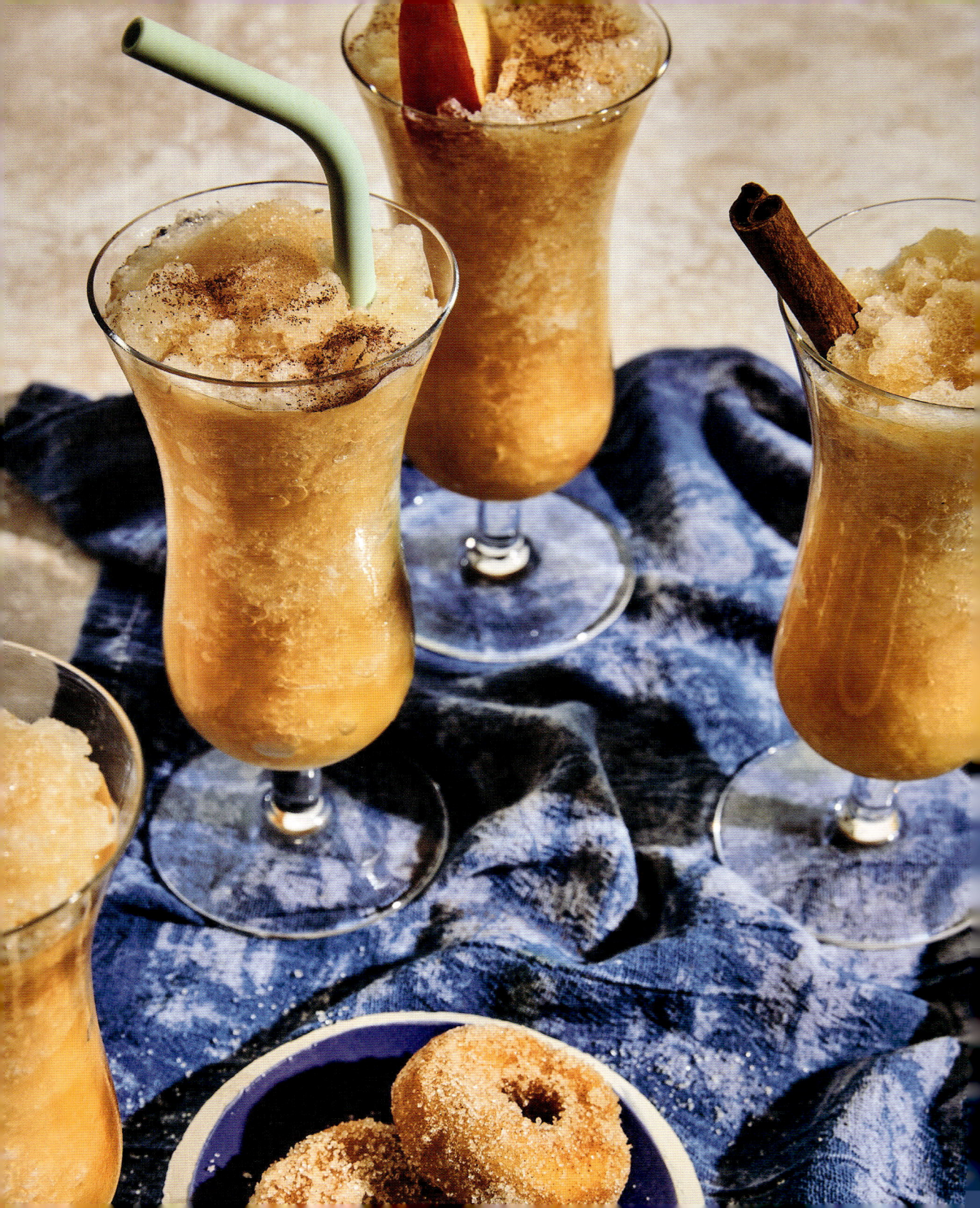

ORCHARD *Freeze*

SERVES 1

1 cup apple cider

½ cup coconut water

Juice of 1 lemon

GARNISH

1½ teaspoons agave syrup

1½ teaspoons ground cinnamon

1½ teaspoons sugar

1 apple slice

Cinnamon stick

Cider donut (optional)

1. Pour the apple cider into ice cube trays and place in the freezer until frozen, about 4 hours.

2. To garnish the rim of your glass, place the agave on a small plate. Mix the cinnamon and sugar on another small plate. Dip a lowball or margarita glass in the agave, then roll in the cinnamon sugar and set aside.

3. Place the frozen cider cubes, coconut water, and lemon juice in a blender and blend until smooth. (You may need to stir and add more coconut water to break down the cubes.)

4. Pour the mixture into the glass and garnish with an apple slice, cinnamon stick, and cider donut (if using) if you want to really bring your own energy.

Every year, I say I'm going apple picking, and every year, life happens and I somehow never make it. But let's be real: I'm mostly in it for the cider and donuts anyway. Orchard Freeze is my way of bringing those cozy and crisp fall flavors to your home—and don't forget the rim inspired by those delicious cider donuts!

HOLIDAY WHO-BEE
What-ee

SERVES 1

½ cup lemon-lime soda

Juice of ½ lime

¼ cup lime sherbert

2 drops green food coloring (optional)

Ice cubes

2 maraschino cherries, for garnish

1. Add the lemon-lime soda and lime juice to a lowball glass.

2. Add the sherbert and food coloring (if using). Stir to combine.

3. Add some ice cubes and top with the cherries.

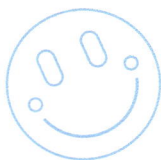

If there's one thing I love, it's The Grinch. I quote it year-round like it's a personality trait. So naturally, I had to create a drink worthy of Whoville itself. This festive lime drink is as green and jolly as the Grinch (post–heart growth, of course).

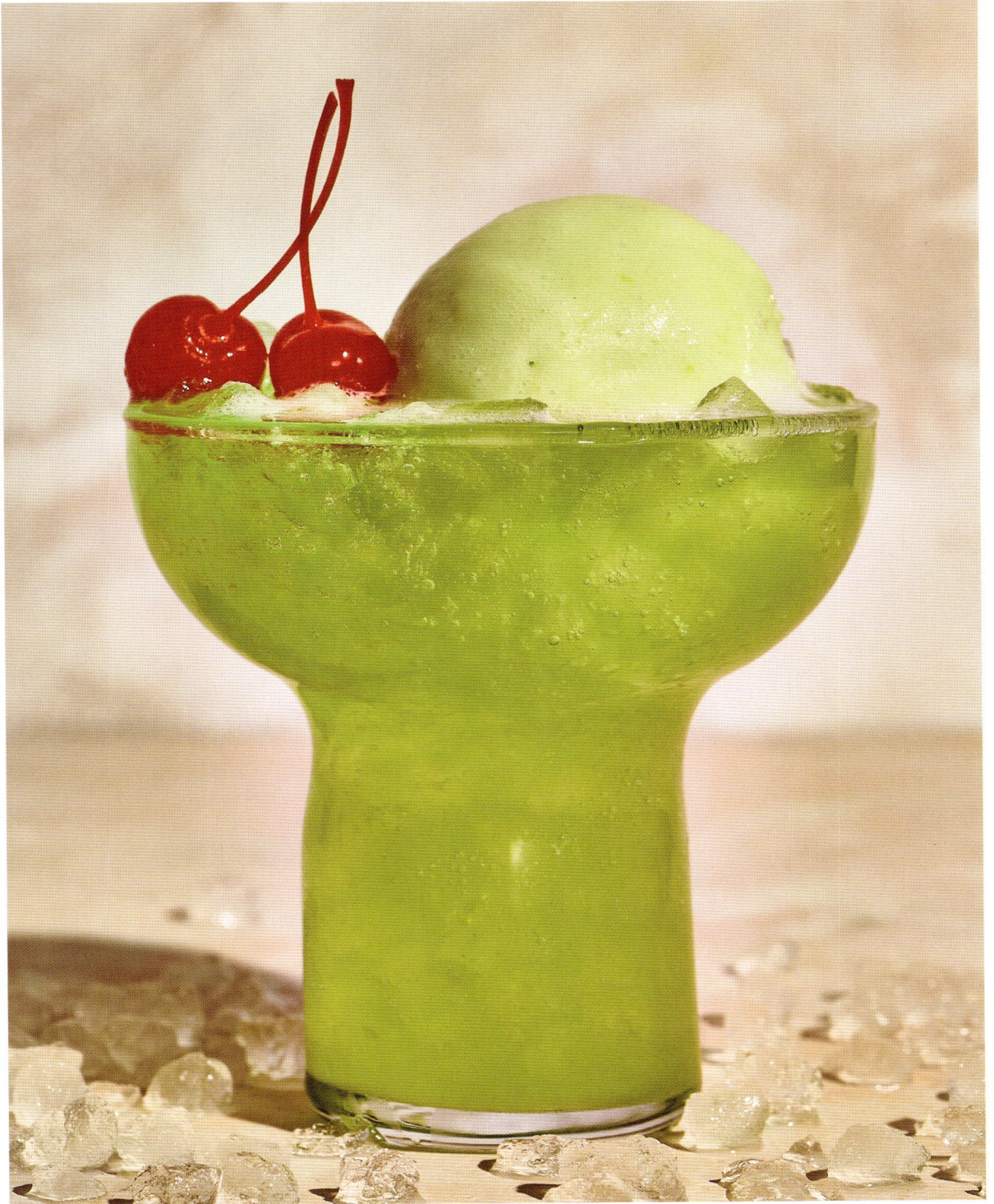

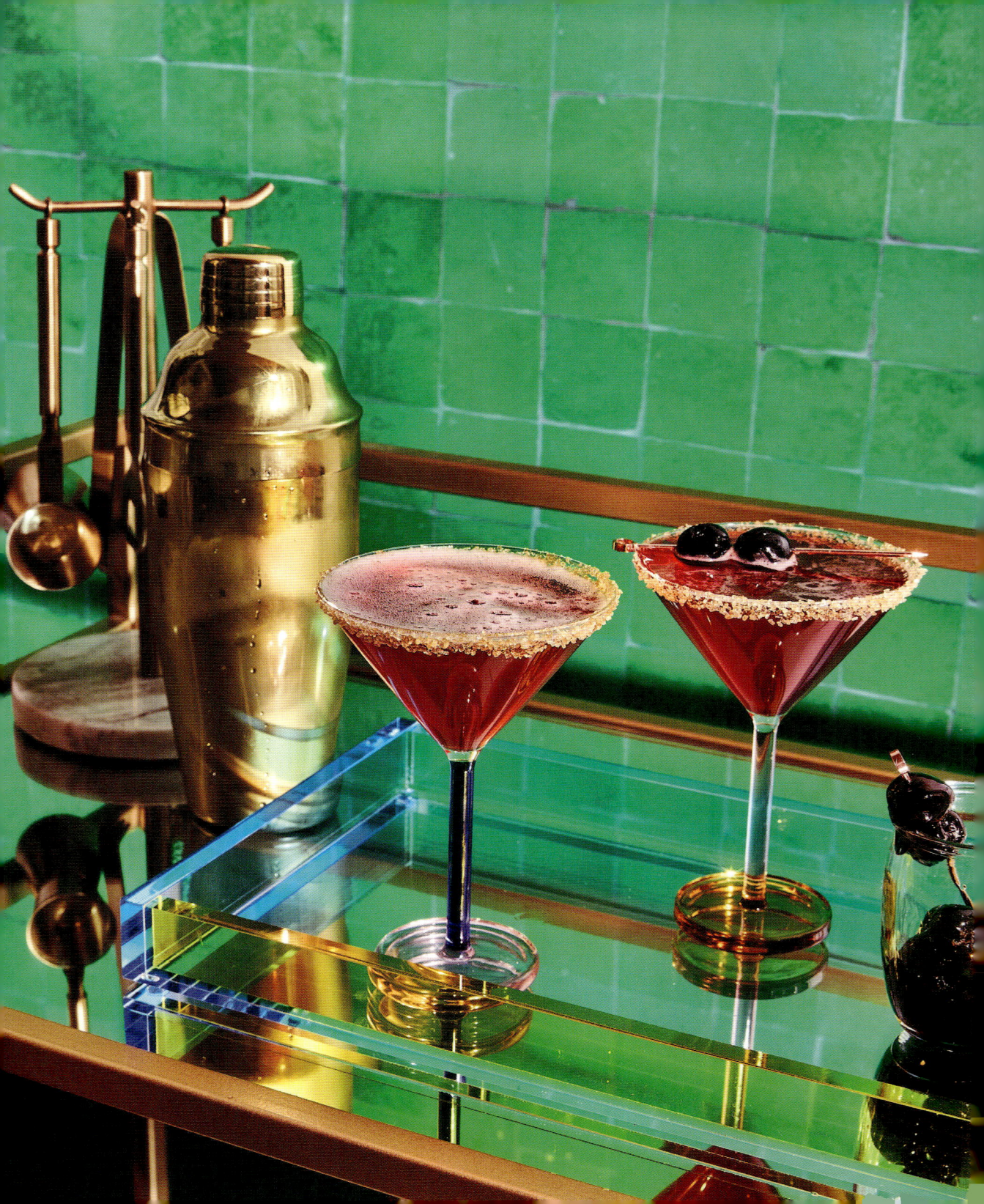

CRANBERRY COSMOPOLITAN

CAROLS
& Cosmos

SERVES 1

⅓ cup unsweetened cranberry juice

2 tablespoons orange juice

Juice of ½ lime

Ice cubes

2 tablespoons sparkling water

GARNISH

1 lime wedge

1½ teaspoons sugar

2 frozen cranberries

1 rosemary sprig

1. To garnish the rim of your glass, rub a lime wedge around edge of a martini glass. Place the sugar on a small plate, then dip the rim into the sugar to coat.

2. Add the cranberry juice, orange juice, and lime juice to a shaker with a handful of ice. Shake until the outside is frosty, about 15 seconds.

3. Strain the mixture into the glass and top with sparkling water. Garnish with cranberries and a rosemary sprig.

Carols and Cosmos is pure holiday magic: festive, sparkly, and just a little fancy. This drink is perfect to sip on while toasting with friends or wrapping presents solo. Is singing off-key to Mariah and living my best Hallmark movie life too much? Asking for a friend.

HOW TO
Build Confidence

Positive self-talk: Being kind to yourself makes you more confident. Replace *I can't* with *I'm learning*. Swap *I'm not good at this* for *I'm getting better every time*. Your words shape your mindset, so make them refreshing!

Practice and improve: Confidence isn't instantaneous; it's a stirred, not shaken process. Keep stirring, keep trying, and watch how smoothly things start to blend together.

Try something new: Ever tried a basil leaf in your mocktail? Sometimes a little unexpected twist is exactly what you need (And I have a few in this book for you to try!). The same goes for confidence: Step out of your comfort zone, whether it's a new workout, a brighter outfit, or ordering a mocktail for the first time.

Set small goals and celebrate: Even the tiniest achievement deserves a little flair. Set small, achievable goals and celebrate when you crush them.

Speak your mind: Confidence isn't about being the loudest in the room; it's about knowing that your voice matters. Just like sparkling water adds that fizz factor, speaking up adds a sparkle to your personality. Share your thoughts, stand up for yourself, and watch your confidence bubble over.

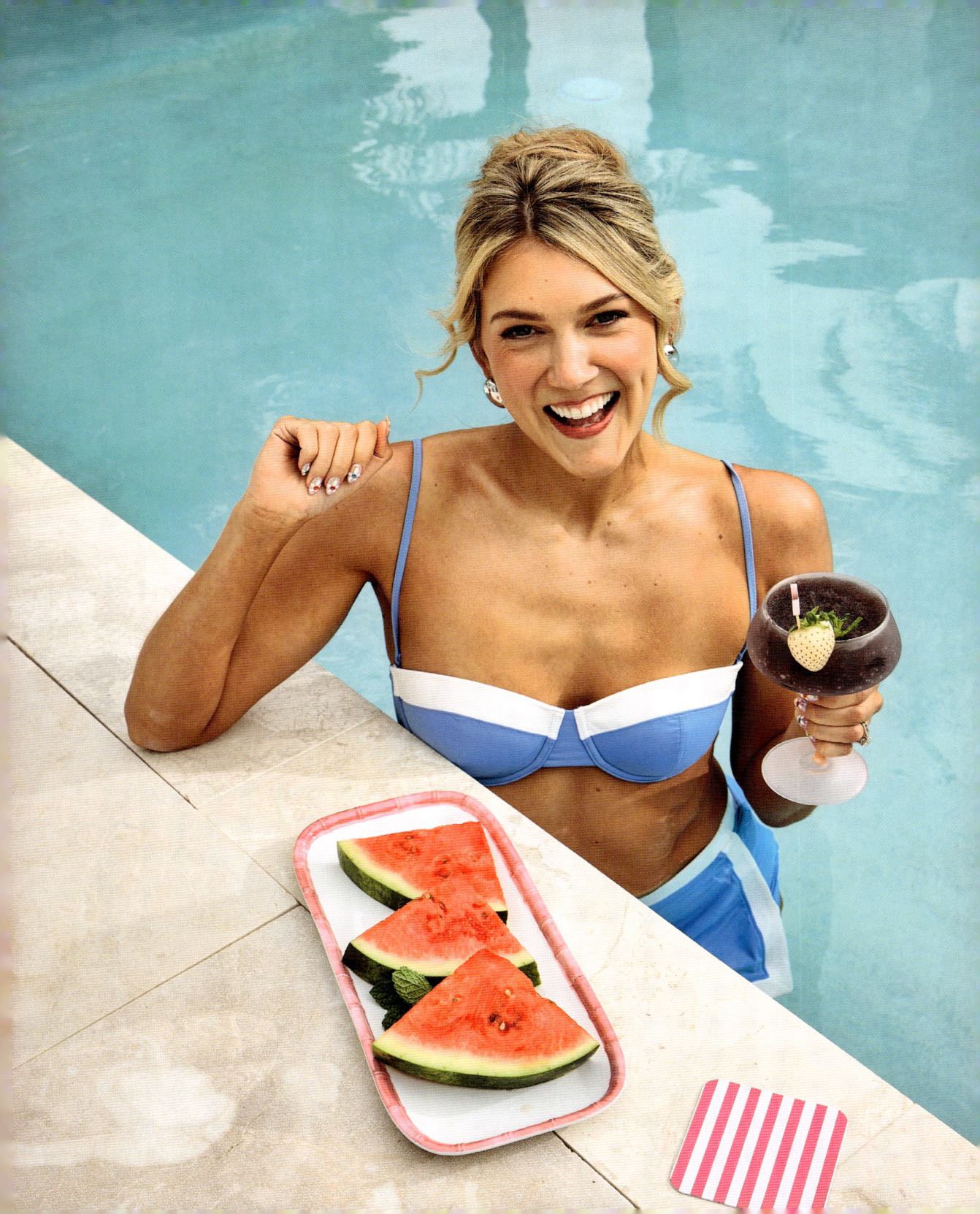

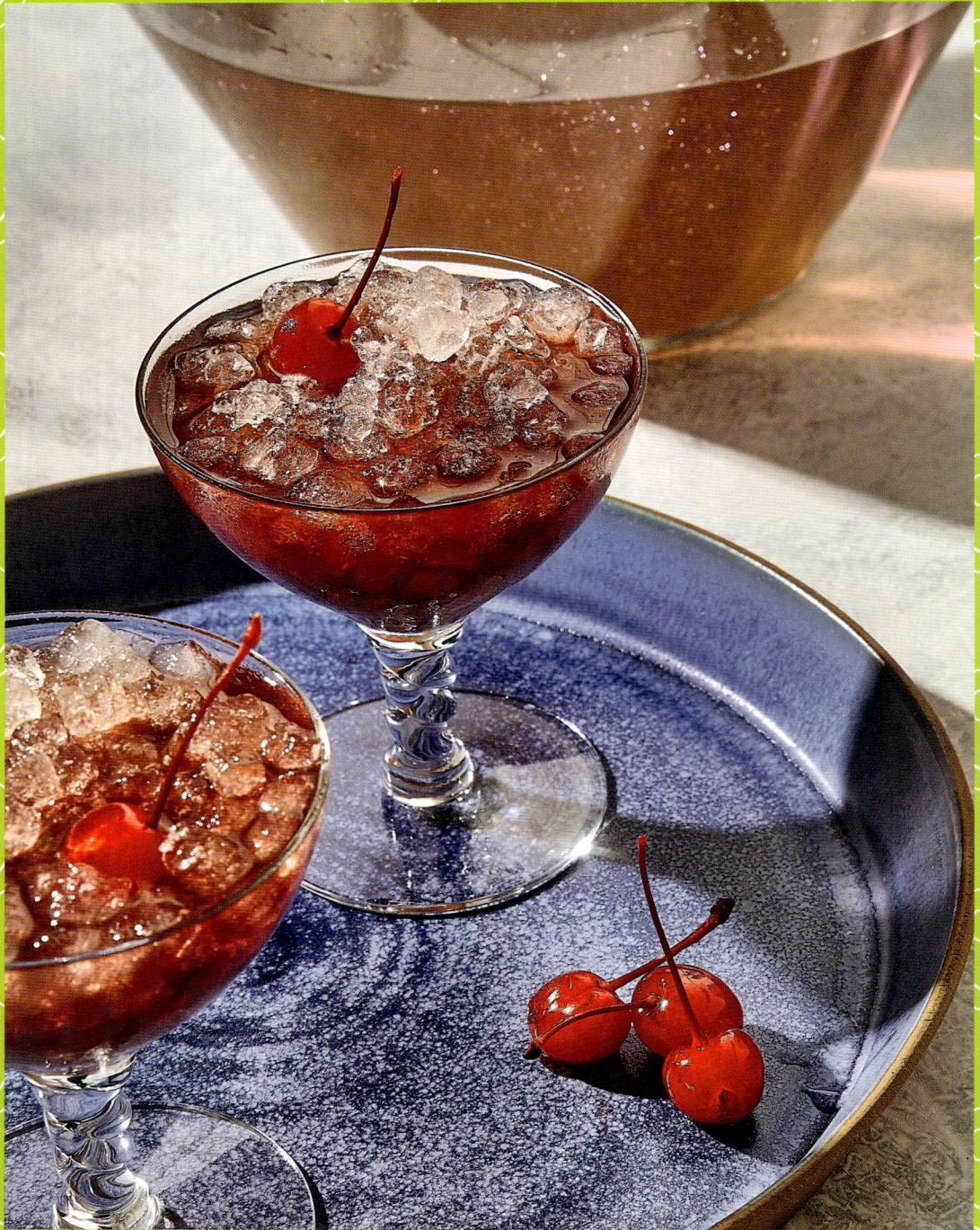

CHAPTER SIX

PARTY
Time

*P*arty time is all about celebrating in style with big-batch mocktails that keep the good times flowing. You can party all night (I'll be in bed by 9, though), enjoy every sip, and wake up feeling fabulous while reminiscing on all the good times you've had.

SIP HAPPENS
Sangria

SERVES 8

4 cups green tea, cooled to room temperature

2 cups white grape juice

½ cup orange juice

½ cup honey (optional)

1 cup diced pineapple

1 peach, pitted and sliced

2 plums, pitted and sliced

½ cup unflavored sparkling water

Ice cubes

1. Combine the green tea, grape juice, and orange juice in a large pitcher or bowl.

2. Add the honey (if using) and stir until dissolved.

3. Add the pineapple, peach, and plums.

4. Cover and let sit for at least 2 hours. (I always end up putting this in the refrigerator 3 hours before guests arrive.)

5. When you're ready to serve, top with sparkling water and stir. Serve the sangria over ice and enjoy.

TIP If using a dispenser, consider having cut-up fruit for guests to garnish their drinks with since they will be strained.

Life doesn't always go as planned, but that's why we have sangria! Light, crisp, and simply delicious, this sangria is here for the good times, the moments you want to purposefully forget, and everything in between. So when life gives you lemons, or a fridge full of fruit, just remember, sip happens!

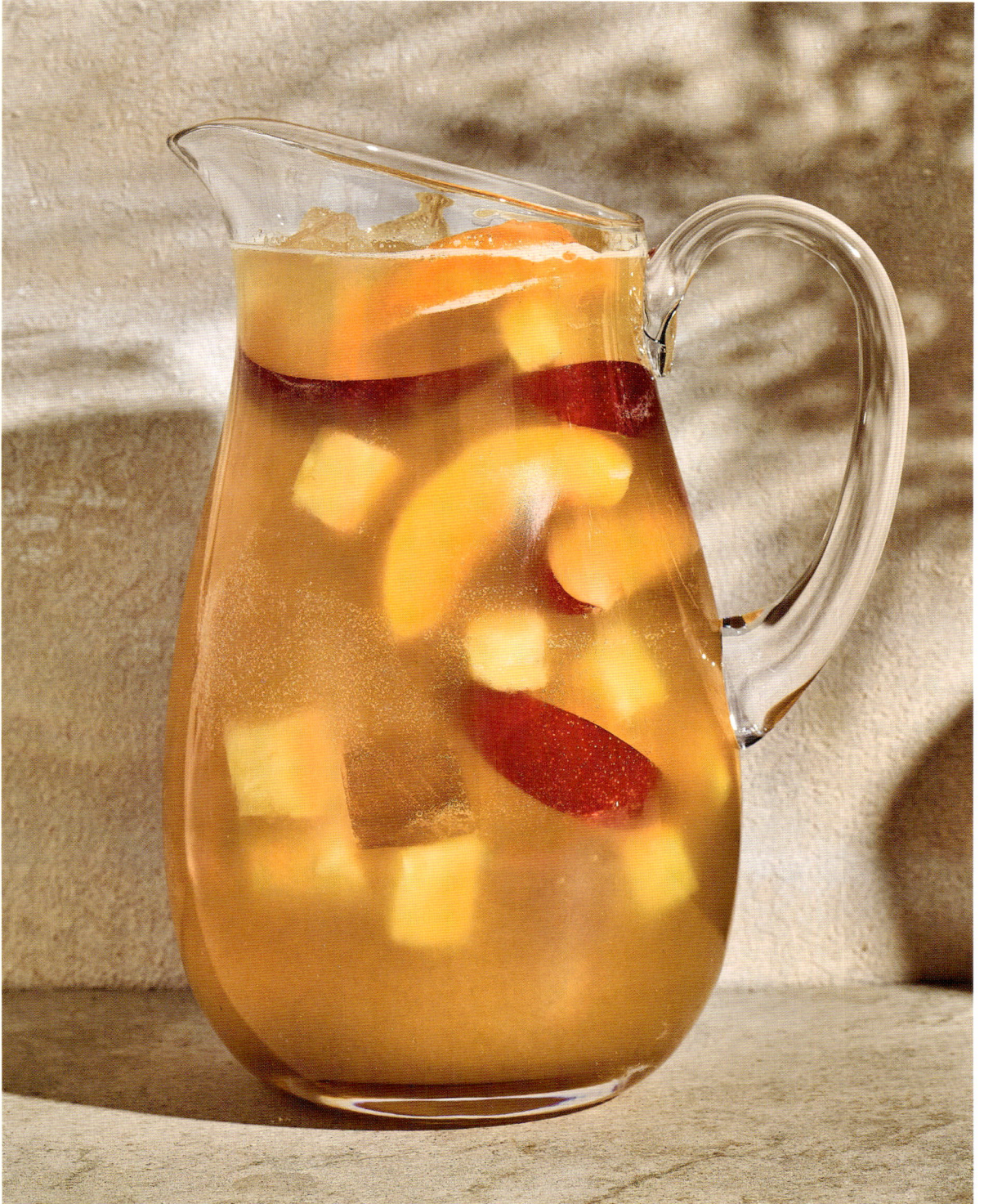

LAVENDER HAZE *Punch*

SERVES 8

8 cups water

Juice of 8 lemons

2 cups lavender syrup

3 to 5 drops purple food coloring (optional)

1 teaspoon edible glitter (optional)

Ice cubes

1. Add the water, lemon juice, lavender syrup, food coloring (if using), and glitter (if using) to a punch bowl. Fill with ice and stir.

2. Ladle into glasses and serve.

This punch right here is one of my faves for many reasons, and you can probably guess why. The lavender and lemon combo will make you romanticize your life, and I love that for you. Belt out your favorite song, twirl in the kitchen, or vibe in your comfiest sweats while sipping on this—and boom, you'll be in your soft, sparkly no-drama era.

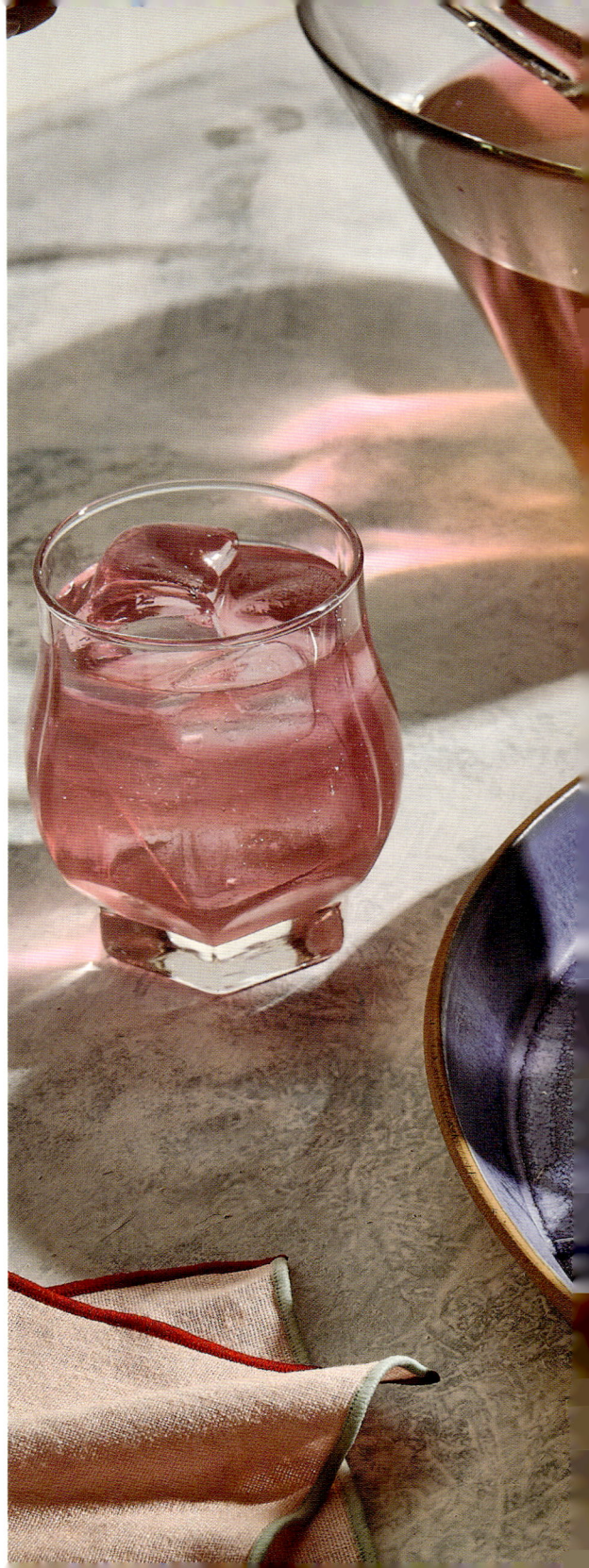

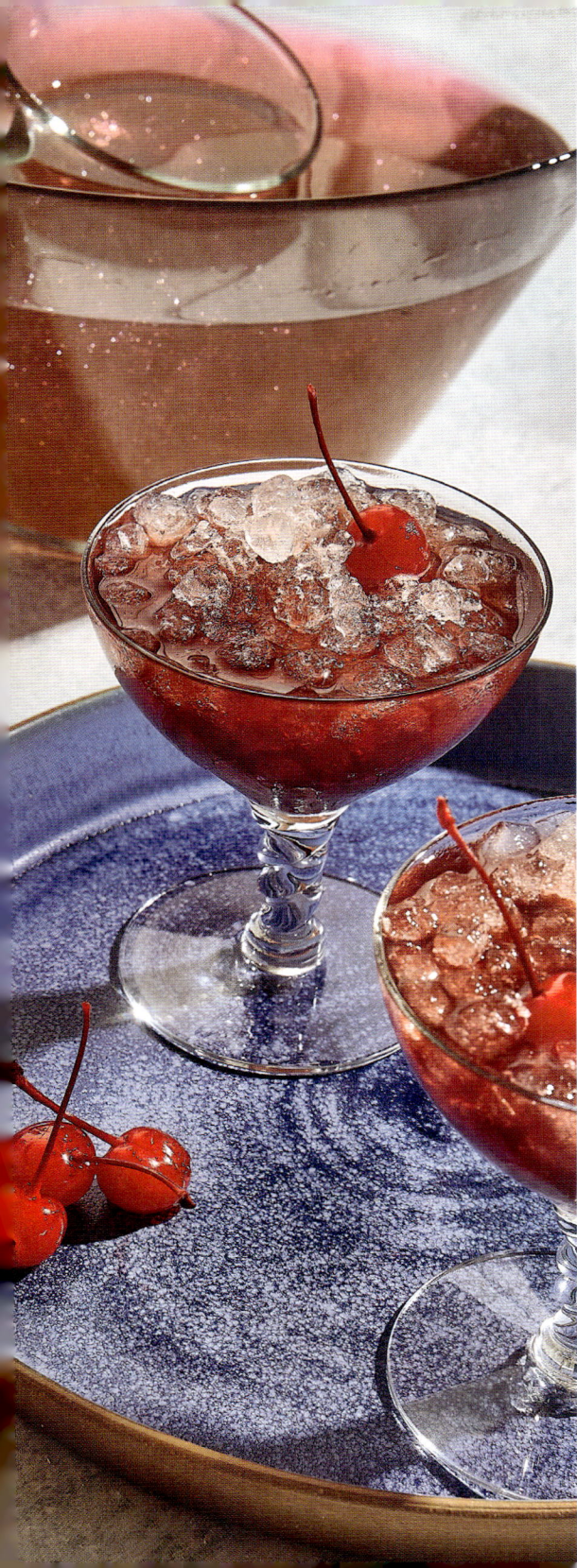

CHERRY LIME
& Unwind

SERVES 8

3½ cups unflavored or lime sparkling water

2 cups tart cherry juice

Juice of 8 limes

½ cup agave syrup

Nugget ice or mini ice cubes from tray molds (optional)

1. Combine the sparkling water, cherry juice, lime juice, and agave in a large pitcher and stir.

2. When ready to serve, fill lowball glasses with nugget ice (if using) and pour in the drinks.

Who remembers Sonic Cherry Limeade with the nugget ice? Did the servers at Sonic wear roller skates, or am I making that up? Anyhoo, I was determined to make a similar drink with a lot less sugar and way more benefits. Tart cherry juice not only helps you sleep but is great for decreasing inflammation and boosting brain function. If this drink doesn't take you back in time, then shucks.

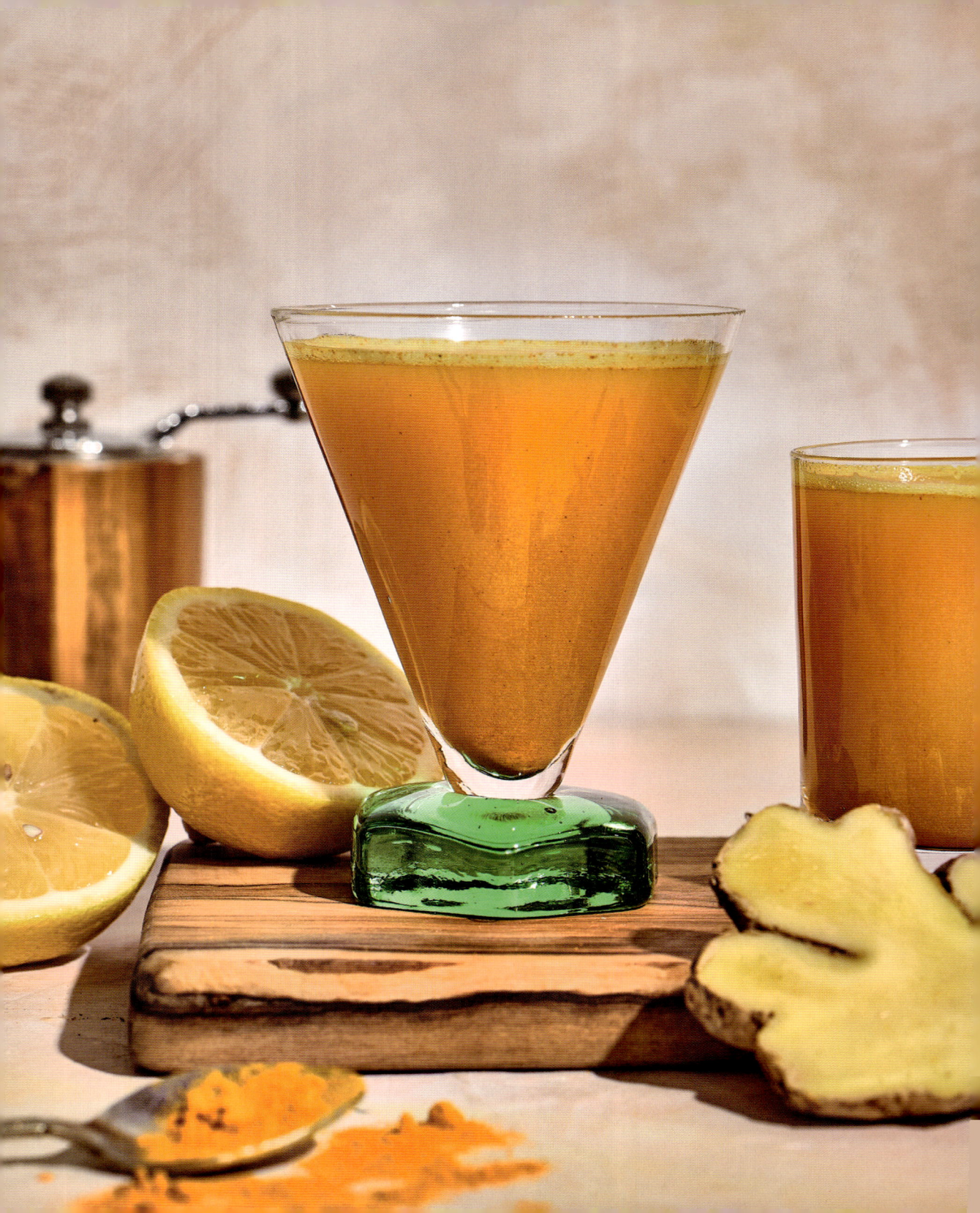

FOREVER *Young*

SERVES 8

One 6 to 8-inch piece ginger, peeled

4 cups water

Juice of 6 to 8 lemons

¼ cup honey

2 teaspoons cayenne

2 teaspoons ground turmeric

1 teaspoon black pepper

1. Add the ginger, water, lemon juice, honey, cayenne, turmeric, and black pepper to a blender. Blend until the ginger is fully broken down.

2. Strain the mixture through a fine-mesh strainer or nut milk bag into a bowl.

3. Divide the mixture among shot glasses and enjoy.

Forever Young is a spicy reset button in a shot glass. These wake up those taste buds and your immune system. After I down one of these, I feel like I just did a strength workout, took a power nap, and made a really responsible life choice. It's not quite the fountain of youth, but hey, it's close enough.

MINTY *Mules*

SERVES 8

2 cups mint leaves

Juice of 4 limes

Ice cubes

8 cups ginger beer, chilled

1. Place the mint leaves and lime juice in a pitcher and muddle until fragrant, about 5 twists.

2. Fill the pitcher halfway with ice if desired (or you can fill individual cups with ice).

3. Top with ginger beer and stir. Serve immediately.

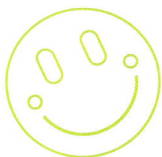

When the party is going strong, the last thing you want to do is play bartender all night. And that's where Minty Mule comes in. The cooling mint, zesty lime, and bold ginger end up being the life of the party. So pour yourself a glass and enjoy, because this drink can stir itself.

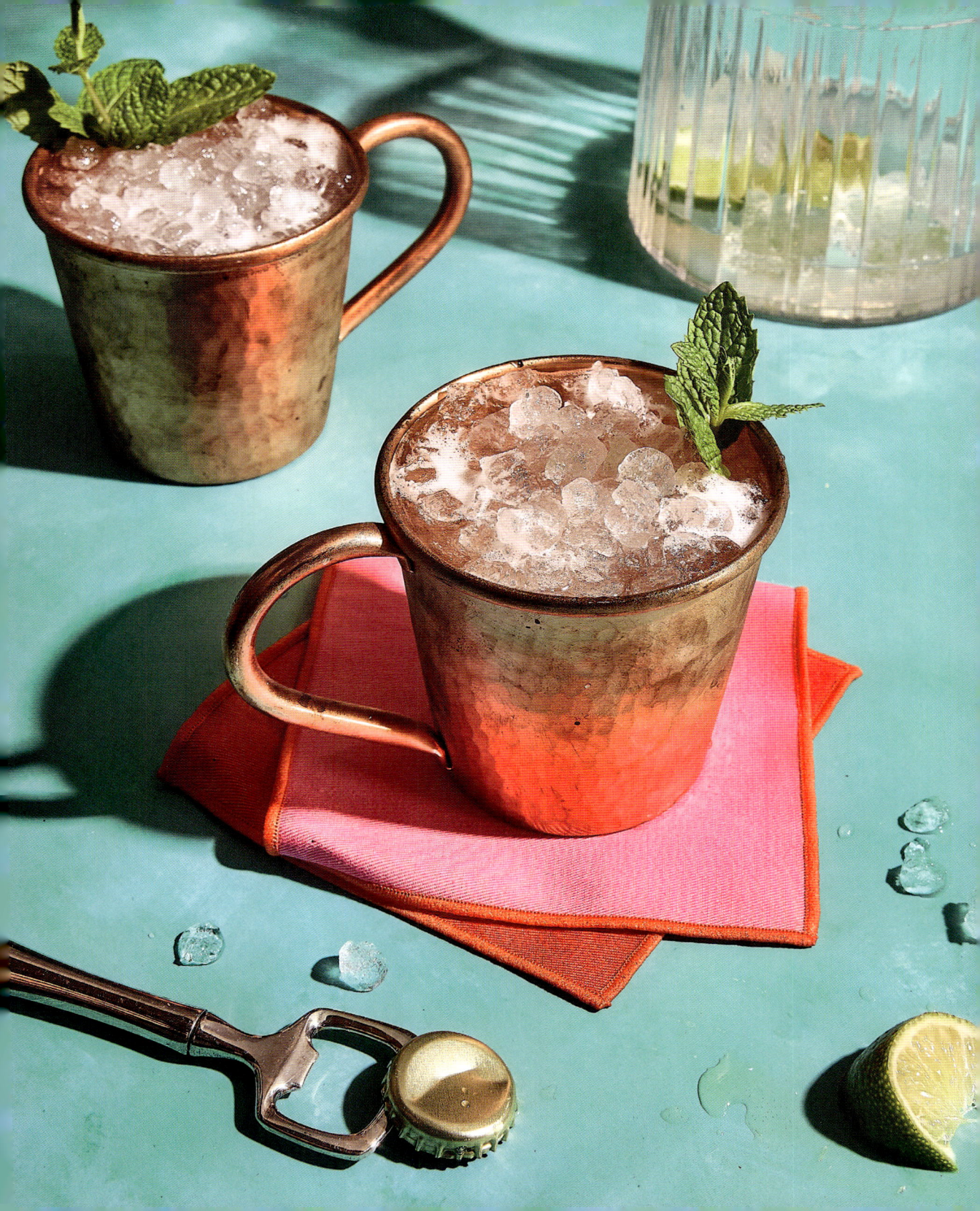

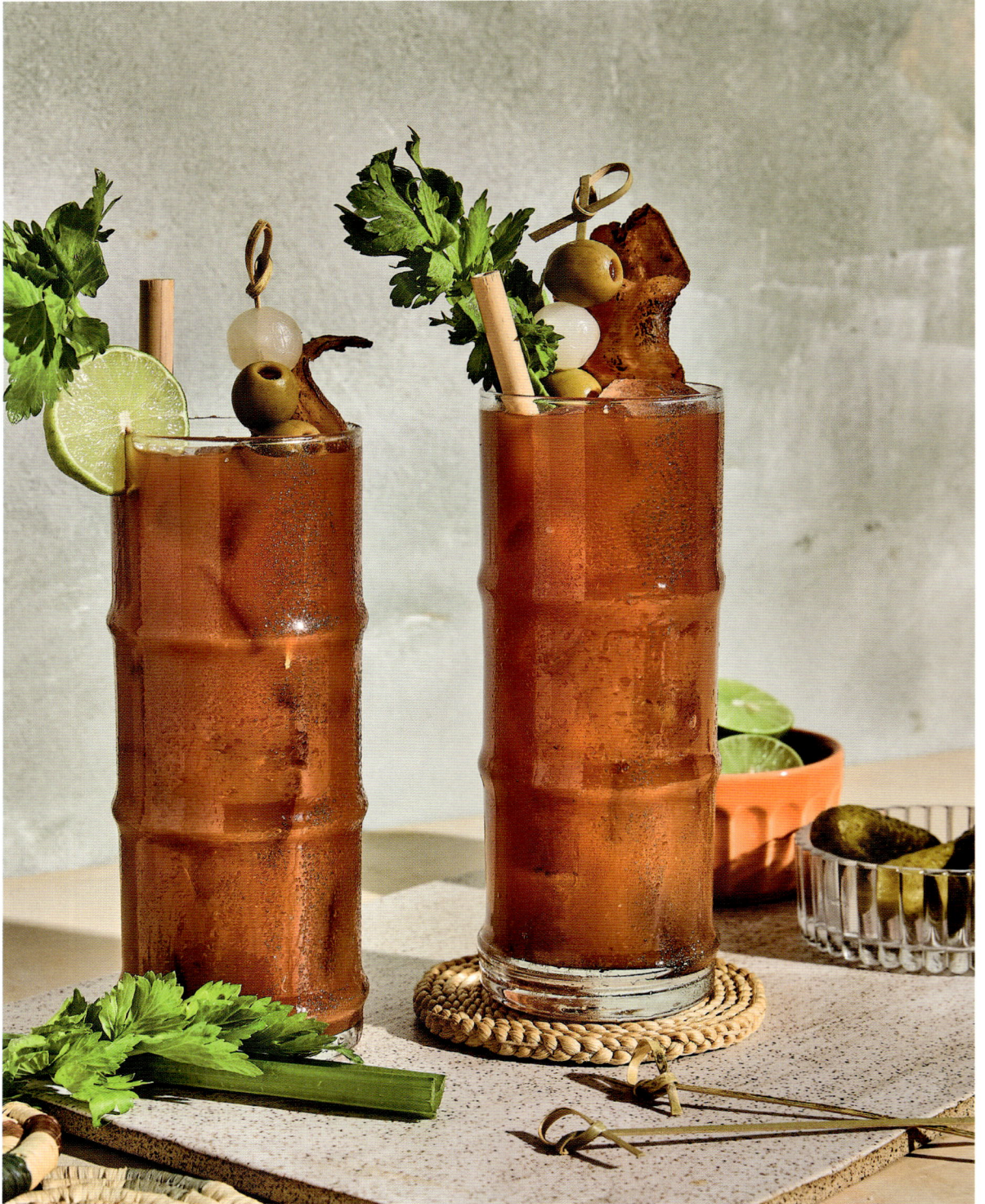

STRONG LIKE *Mary*

SERVES 8

8 cups tomato juice (I like low-sodium)

Juice of 4 lemons

½ cup pickle juice, from a pickle jar (I like Wickles Pickles)

4 teaspoons hot sauce

2 teaspoons Worcestershire sauce

2 teaspoons prepared horseradish

2 teaspoons black pepper, or to taste

2 teaspoons celery salt, or to taste

Ice cubes

GARNISH

Bacon slices

Celery stalks

Lime rounds

Pearl onions

Pickle spears

1. Place the tomato juice, lemon juice, pickle juice, hot sauce, Worcestershire sauce, horseradish, black pepper, and celery salt in a large pitcher and stir thoroughly.

2. Set in the fridge for at least 3 hours to let the flavors combine.

3. To serve, fill tall glasses with ice and pour in the drinks. Add your favorite garnishes (see Tip).

Strong Like Mary isn't just a mocktail; it's a reminder that strength is within all of us. With bold, savory flavors, this drink is about embracing your inner power and finding strength to transform your life. Sip this and remember that being strong like Mary can change everything.

TIP Set out a garnish station so guests can pick their favorites and add them to their drinks!

SPICED & NICE
Cider

SERVES 8

10 pears, quartered

1 orange, sliced

2 cups cranberries

4 cinnamon sticks

12 whole cloves

1 whole nutmeg

8 cups water

½ cup agave syrup

GARNISH

Apple slices

Cranberries

Orange slices

Cinnamon sticks

1. Add the pears, orange slices, cranberries, cinnamon sticks, cloves (see Tip), and nutmeg to a slow cooker.

2. Add the water, then turn the slow cooker to low and cook for 4 to 5 hours, so the fruits and spices can infuse the liquid.

3. One hour before the cider is ready, mash the fruits together to release all the flavors and juices. Strain the mixture through a fine-mesh sieve into a large bowl. Discard the fruit.

4. Rinse the slow cooker, then return the strained cider back to the slow cooker. Add the agave and stir.

5. Serve with the garnishes displayed near the cups so everyone can choose how they wish to garnish their cider.

TIP I like to stick the cloves into the orange slices, so they release their flavor gradually. This prevents the clove flavor from being too overpowering.

There is nothing cozier than a drink that does all the work for you. This is the ultimate set-it-and-forget-it recipe, filling your house with a dreamy aroma as it simmers away in the crockpot. It's perfect for chilly nights, holiday gatherings, or just because you deserve something warm and wonderful. No slow cooker? Just use a large pot on the stovetop.

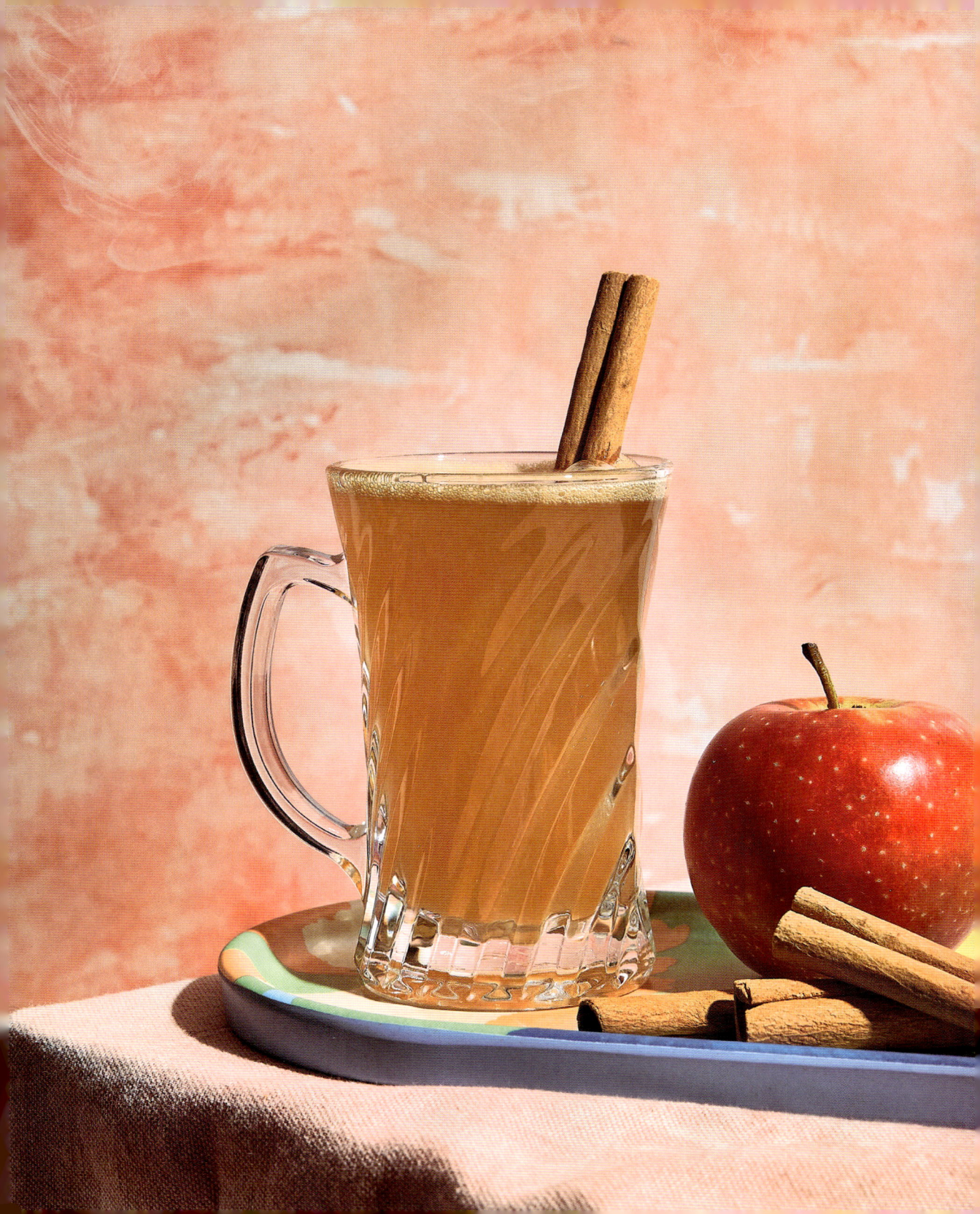

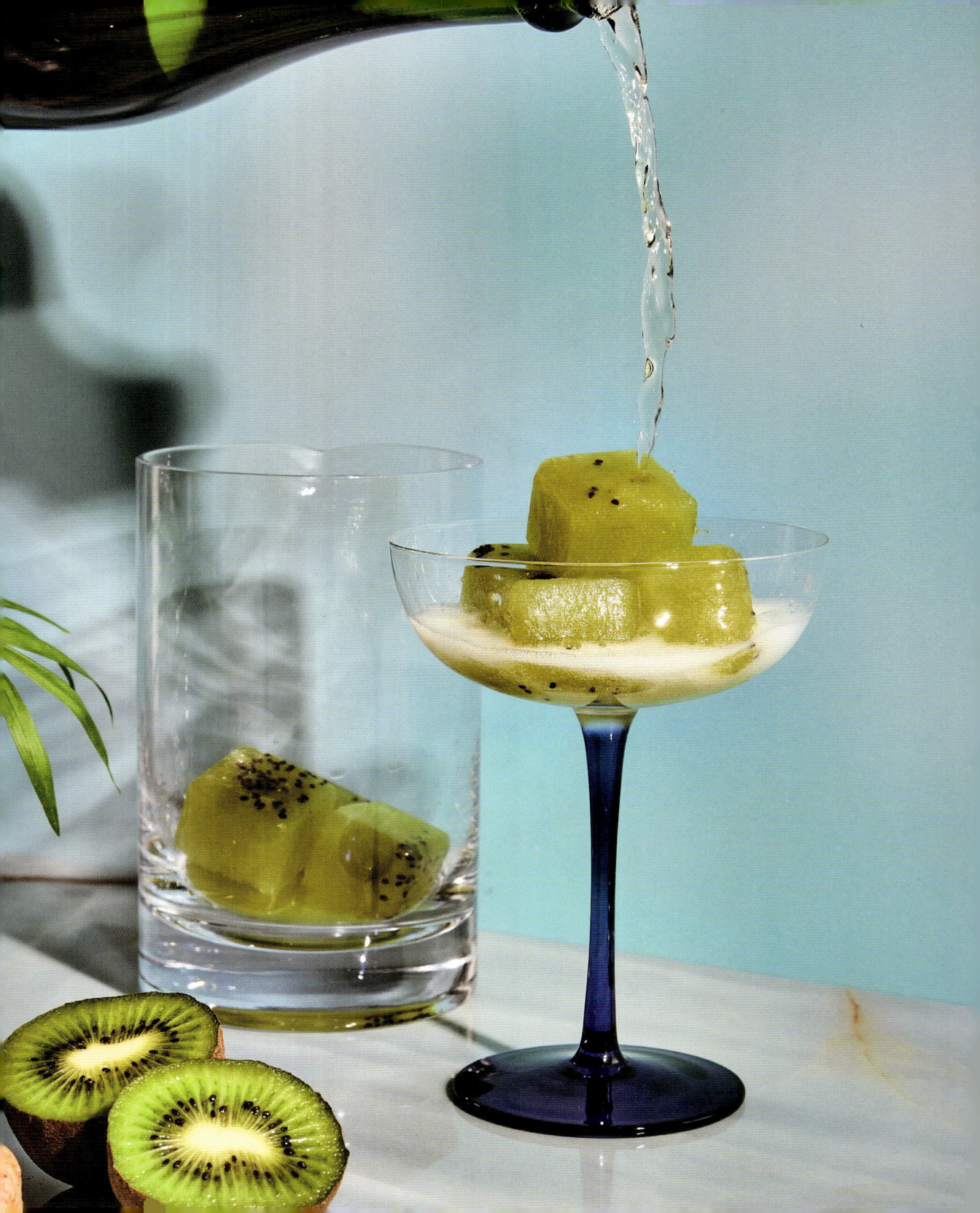

BELLINI ME, *Please*

SERVES 8

8 kiwis, peeled and chopped

Juice of 1 lime

¼ cup agave syrup

One 750 ml bottle alcohol-removed brut champagne (I like Fre; see Note 1)

1. Place the kiwis, lime juice, and agave in a blender (see Note 2). Blend just until smooth, 15 to 20 seconds. (Don't blend for too long or the mixture will turn brown.)

2. Pour the puree into small ice molds and place in the freezer until frozen, about 5 hours.

3. Place 1 to 4 ice cubes in a coupe glass and top with the champagne.

NOTE 1 Unflavored sparkling water would work here, too!

NOTE 2 You can try different fruits in place of the kiwis and even add mint and lime slices to the molds before freezing, if desired.

Some drinks just get you and Bellini Me, Please is one of them. The juicy kiwi-packed ice cubes fizzing in the alcohol-removed champagne make any moment a celebration. Enjoy these at brunch, at happy hour, or just because you deserve it. Have fun with it and experiment with fruits other than kiwis if you desire!

MARRY ME
Margs

SERVES 8

4 cups ginger lemon kombucha

2⅔ cups orange juice

Juice of 4 limes

¼ cup agave syrup

Ice cubes

GARNISH

Lime wedges

Salt

1. Coat the rims of rocks or margarita glasses with a lime wedge. Pour the salt onto a small plate, then dip the rims into the salt to coat.

2. Add the kombucha, orange juice, lime juice, and agave to a pitcher and stir.

3. Add ice directly to the pitcher or to individual glasses. Pour the margs into the glasses and serve.

Marry Me Margs are the type of drink anyone and everyone will love, so they're perfect for a celebration. This zingy, bubbly mocktail brings together a fiery kick of ginger with the bright zest of lemon and fizzy kombucha, all dressed up with a signature margarita salty rim. One sip and you may just say yes to another round.

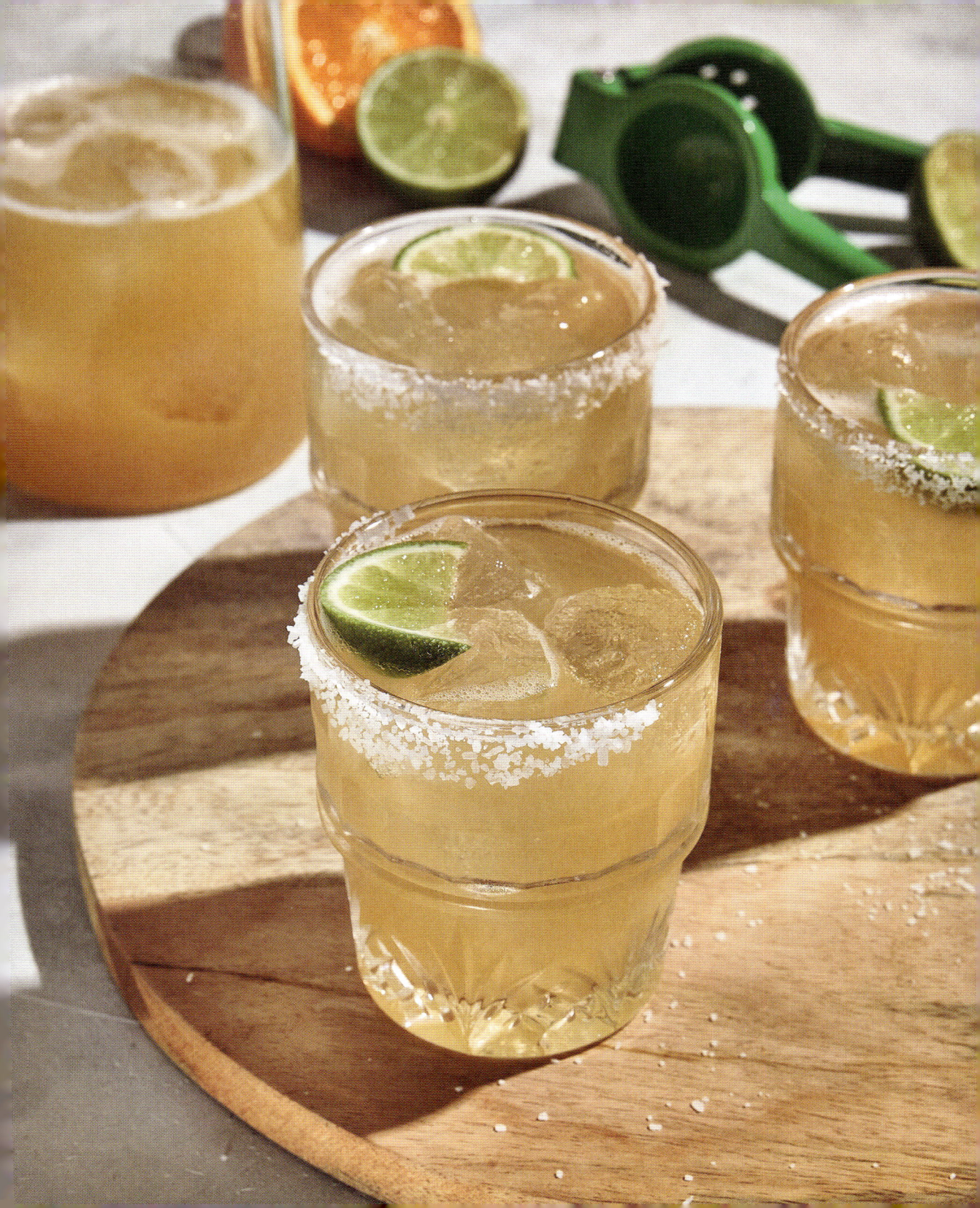

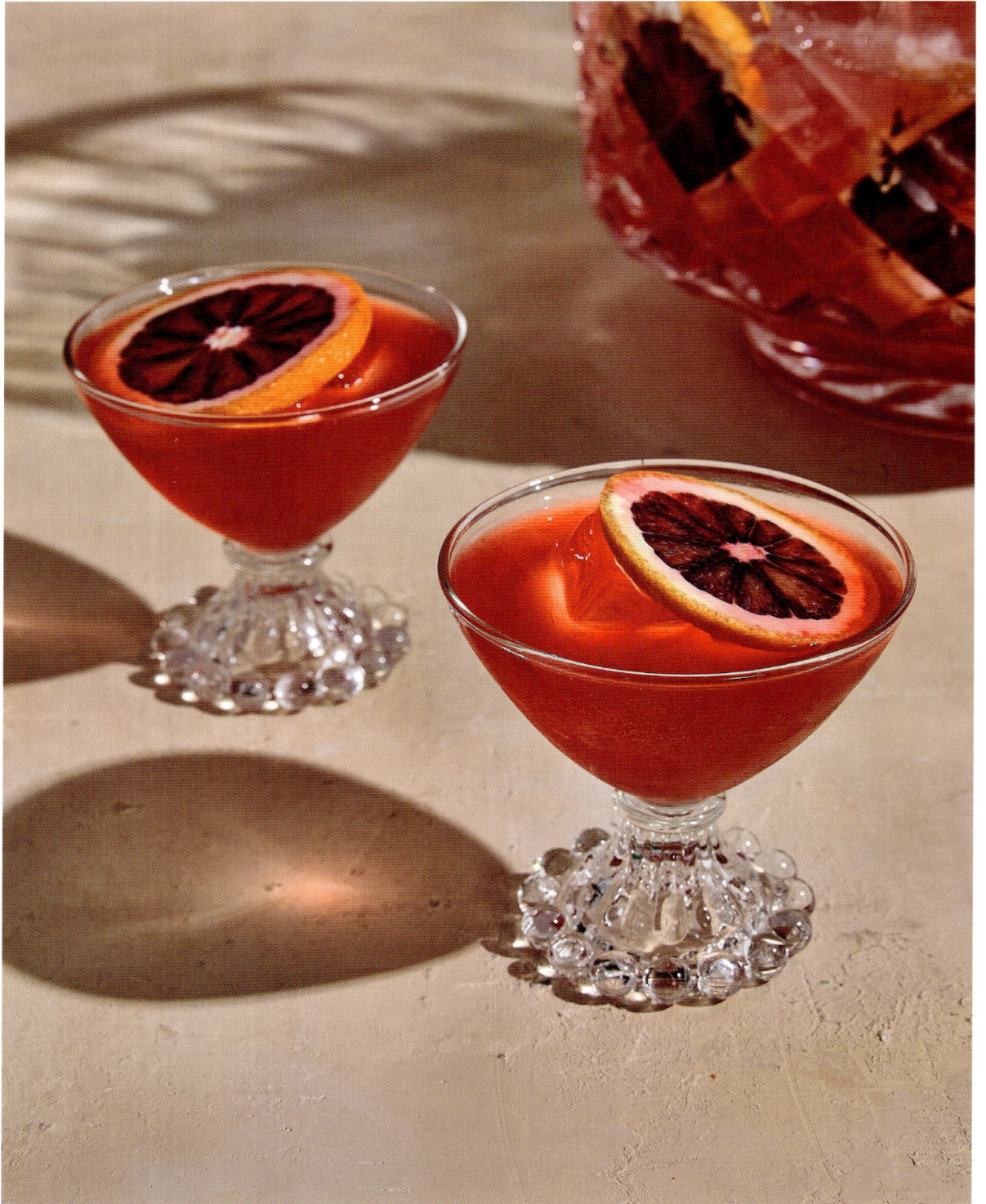

ITALIAN BLOOD ORANGE PUNCH

SING TO ME
Paolo Punch

SERVES 6 TO 8

5 cups Italian blood orange soda (I like Trader Joe's), chilled

½ cup maraschino cherry juice (from a maraschino cherry jar)

Juice of 3 lemons

2 cups unflavored sparkling water, chilled

Ice cubes (optional)

1. Combine the soda, cherry juice, and lemon juice in a punch bowl.

2. Add the sparkling water right before serving to keep the bubbles fresh.

3. Ladle into individual cups, over ice (if using).

This is what dreams are made of—literally! A mocktail even Miss Ungermeyer would approve of. This blood orange punch is as bold and iconic as The Lizzie McGuire Movie *and will transport you to your very own Roman adventure. Grab a glass, channel your inner Lizzie, and have yourself a superstar moment.*

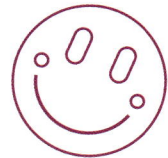

Everyone Will Enjoy

Digital detox night: Unplug and disconnect. Play board games, tell stories, and make your own mocktails.

Gratitude gathering: Have guests share moments of gratitude, write thank you notes, create vision boards, and focus on positive affirmations and intentions.

BYOB: Bring your own board night. Everyone brings a board filled with food: wings board, s'mores board, dip board, candy board, and more. Encourage guests to get creative!

Garden party: Make bouquets and have a seed stand for guests to take home and plant themselves.

Pajama party: Wear your favorite pajamas and watch your favorite 2000s romcom.

Self-care session: Set up self-care stations for skincare, massages, meditations, and stretching.

Journaling and reflection: Create a cozy pillow corner with journals, pens, quotes, and prompts for writing.

DIY craft night: Invite friends over for pottery or jewelry-making.

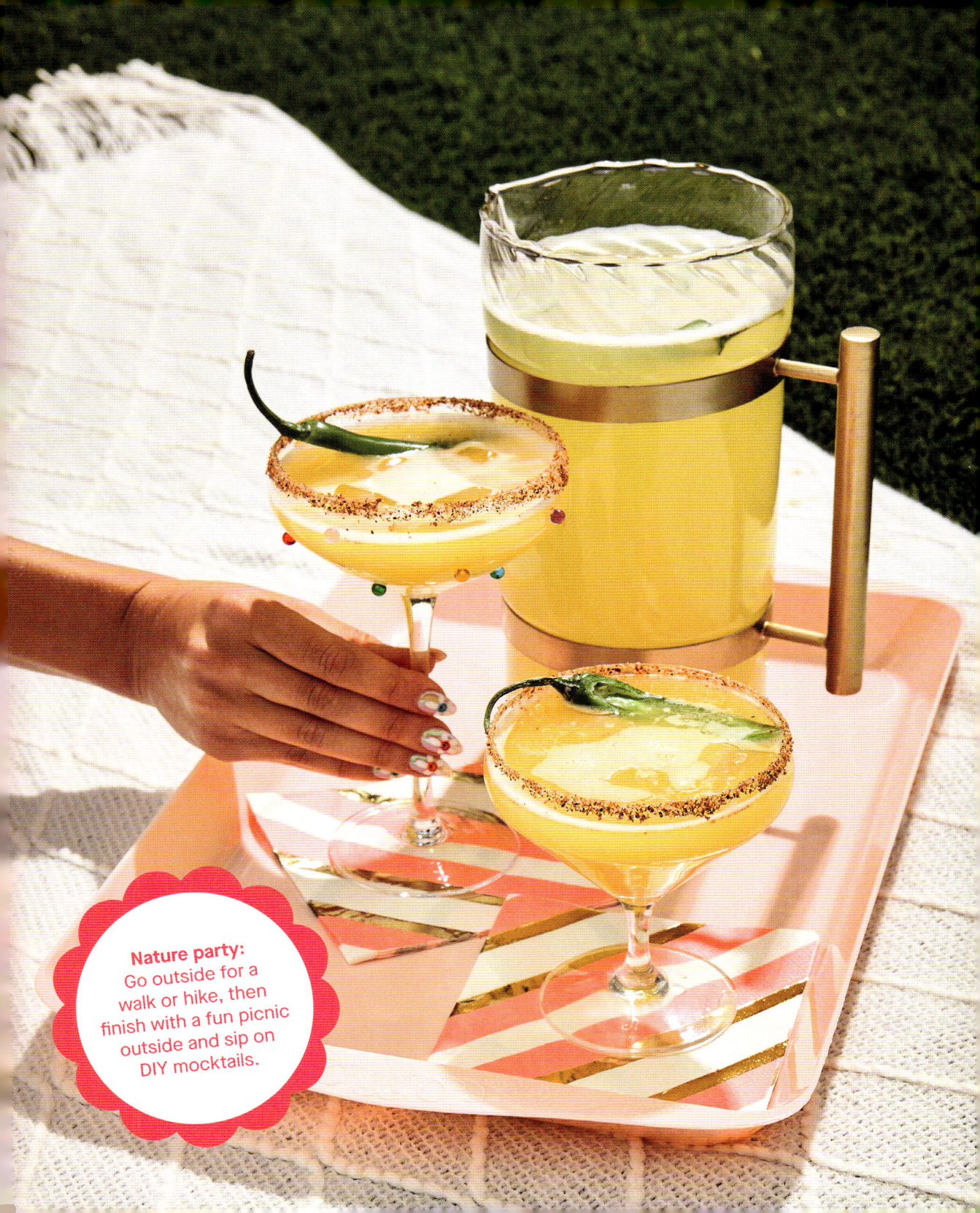

Nature party:
Go outside for a walk or hike, then finish with a fun picnic outside and sip on DIY mocktails.

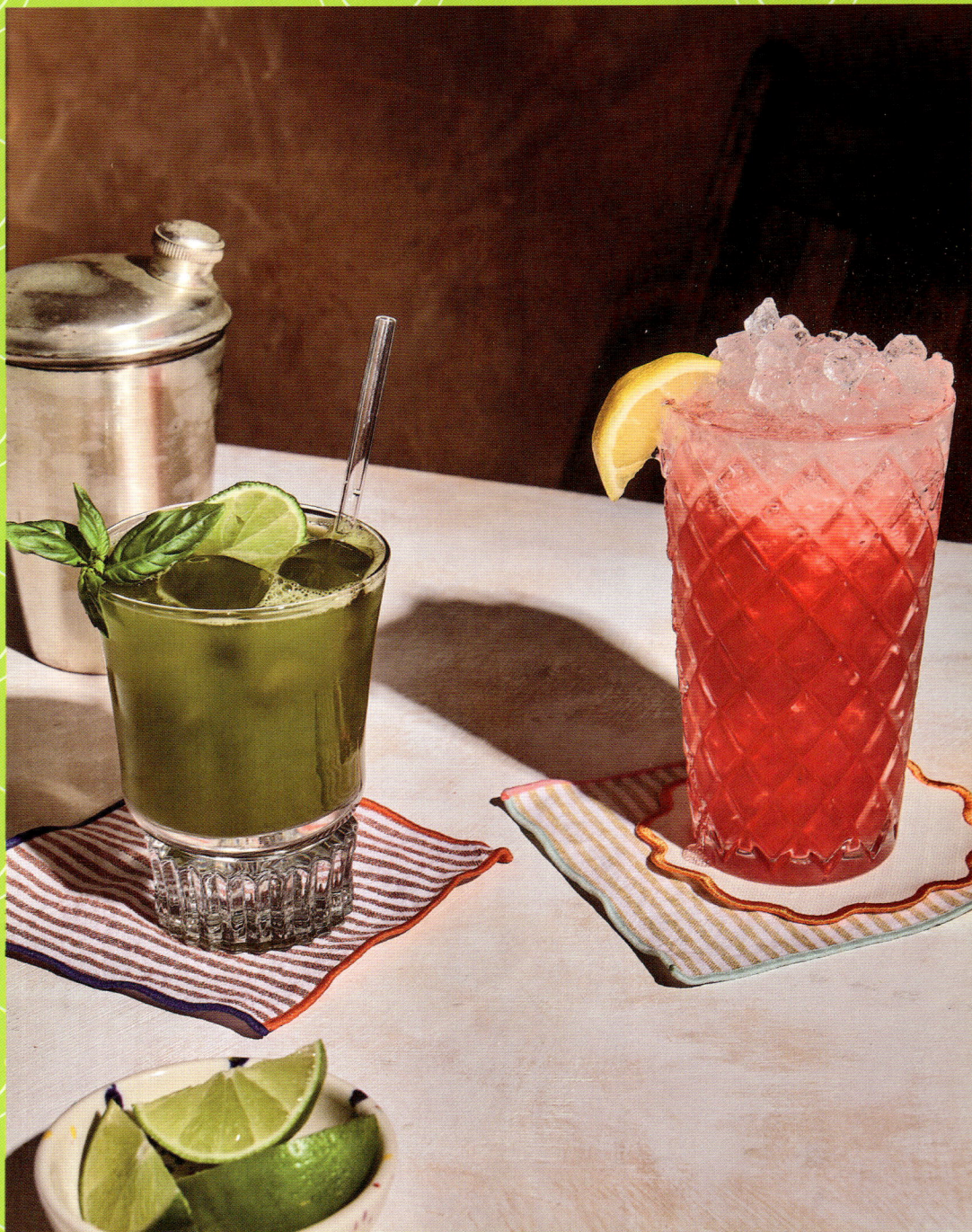

CHAPTER SEVEN

SWEAT, SIP, *Repeat*

Pre- and post-workout mocktails are a thing, and we are here for it. Don't stop at movement; sip your way into wellness with these hydrating, immune-boosting, and refreshing drinks that will leave you feeling great, all day long!

GLOWING
Green

SERVES 1

2 celery stalks, chopped (about ¾ cup)

½ cucumber, chopped (about ¾ cup)

½ green apple, chopped

½ cup water

Juice of ½ lime

Ice cubes

1. Place the celery, cucumber, apple, and water in a blender. Blend until smooth (see Note).

2. Strain the mixture through a fine-mesh strainer (a nut milk bag works best if you have one) over a small bowl.

3. Pour the juice into a lowball glass. Add the lime juice.

4. Fill the glass with ice. Stir and enjoy.

NOTE To make this in a juicer, juice the celery, cucumber, and apple, then pour the juice directly into the glass in step 3.

For the longest time, I tried to be a green juice girlie, but I couldn't find a combination I liked, until I started making it at home. This juice is the ultimate skin-loving, body-refreshing, feel-good drink! The apple adds a touch of sweetness, while the cucumber and celery keep things fresh and detoxifying. This vibrant juice is the perfect way to show your body some love and boost your energy all day long!

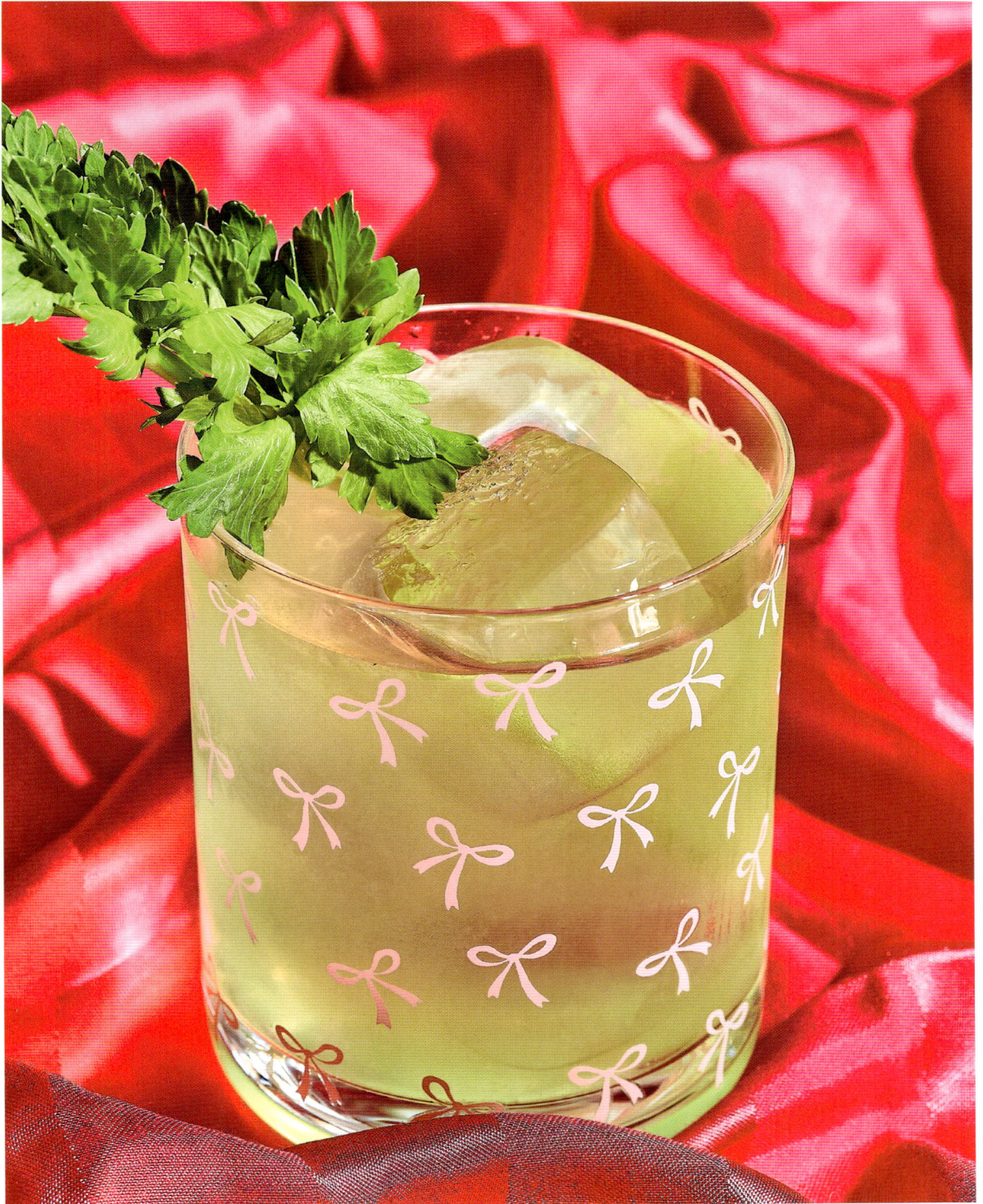

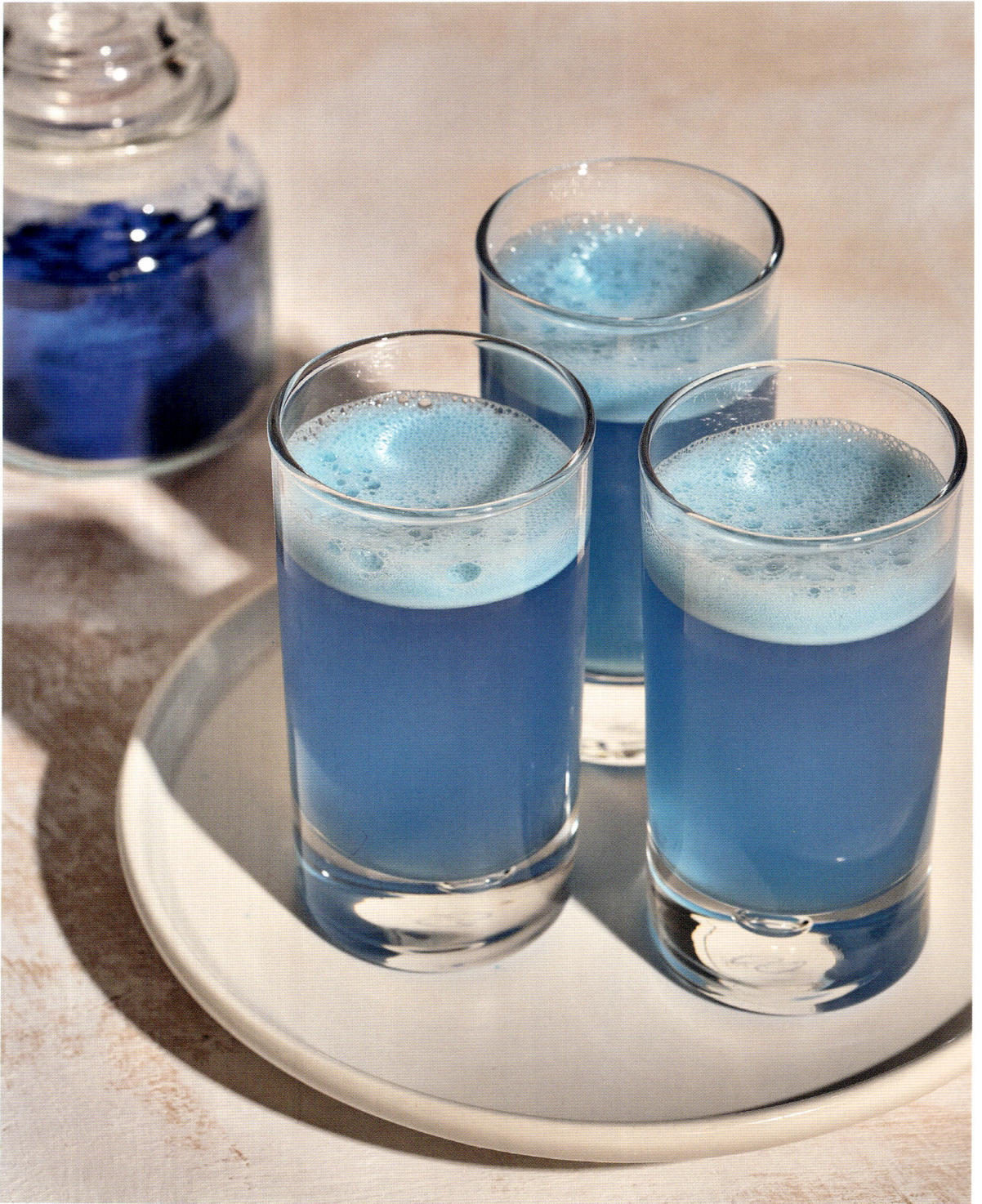

WELLNESS
Wave

SERVES 4

One 2-inch piece ginger, peeled

1 cup coconut water

Juice of 1 lemon

¼ teaspoon blue spirulina powder

1. Place the ginger, coconut water, lemon juice, and spirulina in a blender. Blend until the ginger is fully broken down.

2. Strain the mixture through a fine-mesh strainer or nut milk bag into a bowl.

3. Divide the mixture among shot glasses and serve.

Wellness Wave is like catching the perfect swell—which I have no business even talking about, because I tried to surf once, and the board went straight down into the waves along with me. With spirulina bringing the superfood power, this shot is here to energize, refresh, and maybe even make you feel a little like a health guru (even if your main workout is chasing your kid around). It's bold, bright, and basically the ocean breeze in a bottle.

COOLDOWN
Collins

SERVES 1

1 cup peeled, chopped cucumber

¼ cup coconut water

Ice cubes

Juice of 1 lemon

2 teaspoons agave syrup

1 cup club soda

1. Place the cucumber and coconut water in blender. Blend until smooth.

2. Strain the cucumber puree through a fine-mesh strainer into a shaker.

3. Fill the shaker with a handful of ice, then add the lemon juice and agave.

4. Shake until the outside of the shaker is frosty, about 5 seconds. Fill a Collins glass with ice.

5. Strain the chilled cucumber mixture into the glass. Top with club soda and enjoy.

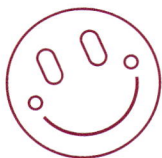

This crisp and cooling Collins mocktail is light and bubbly; it's spa vibes in a cup, which we all could use. Whether you're lounging poolside, need a moment to chill, or are still trying to cool down after your workout, this mocktail is here to keep you calm, cool, and collected.

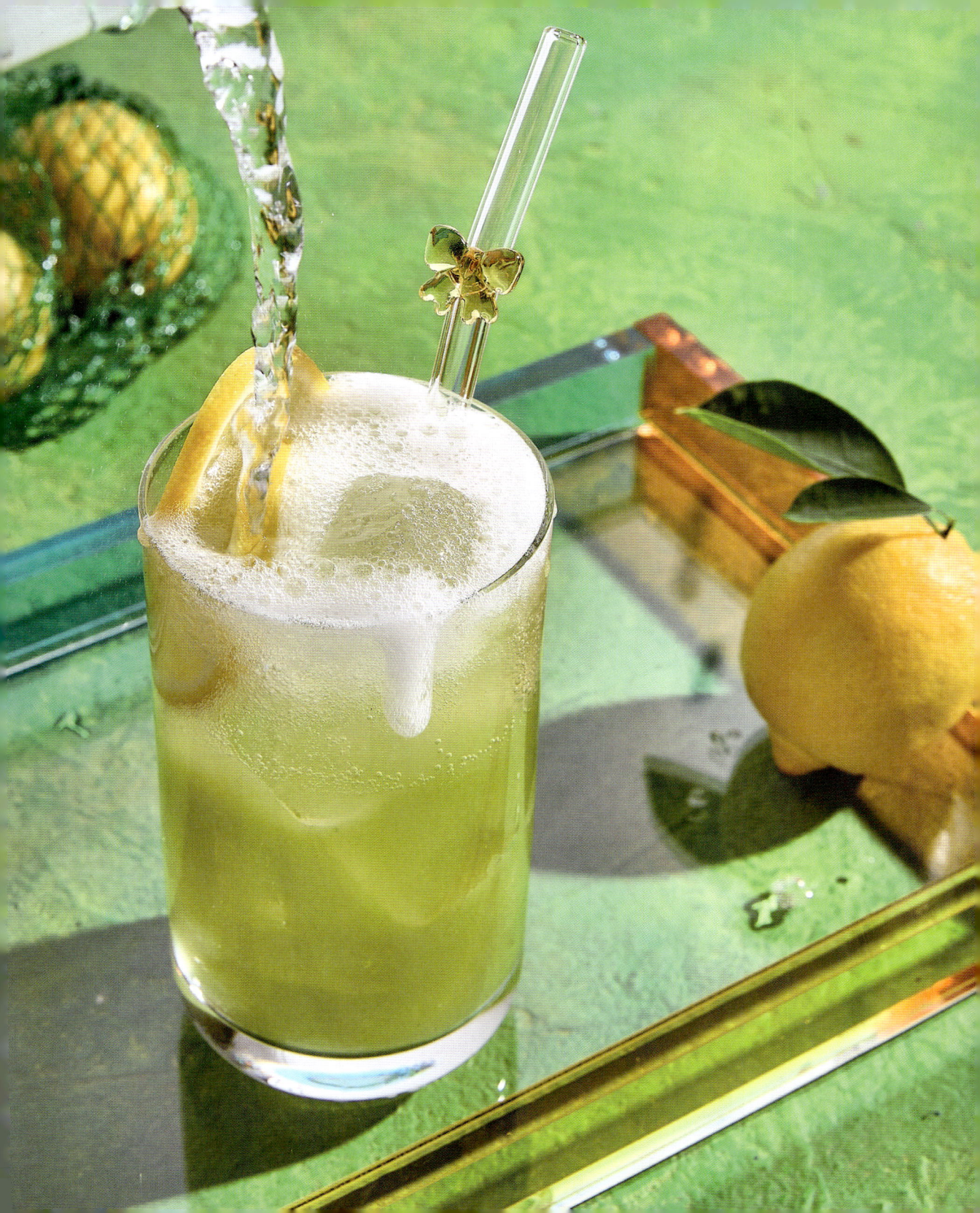

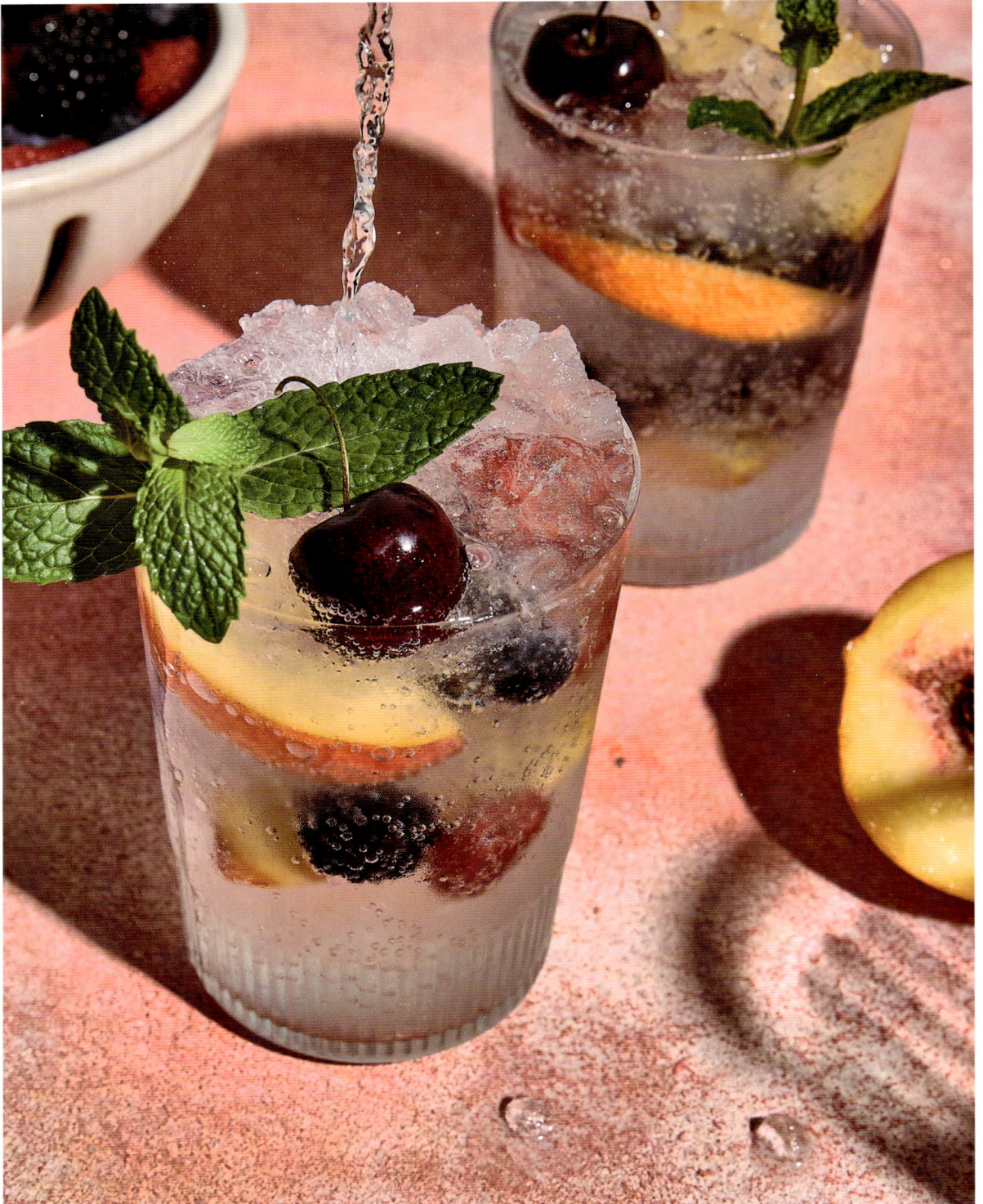

FRUITY COCONUT WATER

IN MY HYDRATION
Era

SERVES 1

Ice cubes

5 raspberries

3 cherries, pitted

5 blueberries

5 blackberries

½ peach, sliced

⅔ cup coconut water

¼ cup coconut seltzer

1 mint sprig, for garnish

1. Place a single layer of ice in the bottom of a lowball glass.

2. Layer your fruit in rainbow order: raspberries, cherries, blueberries, blackberries, and peach slices.

3. Top with more ice, then pour in the coconut water.

4. Top with the seltzer. Garnish with mint (don't forget to clap it between your hands to release its aroma) and enjoy.

In My Hydration Era is the ultimate thirst quencher, packed with juicy fruit and hydrating coconut water. This vibrant drink keeps you refreshed by infusing your water with natural sweetness and nutrients. The best part is that, once you've sipped every last drop, you get to snack on the fruit that has been soaking up all the coconut water. It's hydration and a snack all in one.

RECOVERY
Refresher

SERVES 1

½ cup beet juice

Juice of 1 lemon

1 tablespoon agave syrup

Ice cubes

½ cup coconut water

⅓ cup unflavored sparkling water

1 lemon slice, for garnish

1. Place the beet juice, lemon juice, agave, and a handful of ice in a shaker and shake until the outside is frosty, about 15 seconds.

2. Fill a tall glass with ice and strain the mixture into the glass.

3. Top with coconut water and sparkling water and stir.

4. Garnish with a lemon slice.

After a tough workout or long day, you deserve a drink that works as hard as you do. This Recovery Refresher is packed with powerhouse benefits. Beet juice is known to support stamina, improve blood flow, and help muscles recover, making it the perfect post-sweat sip. It is so delicious, you'll forget it's actually good for you.

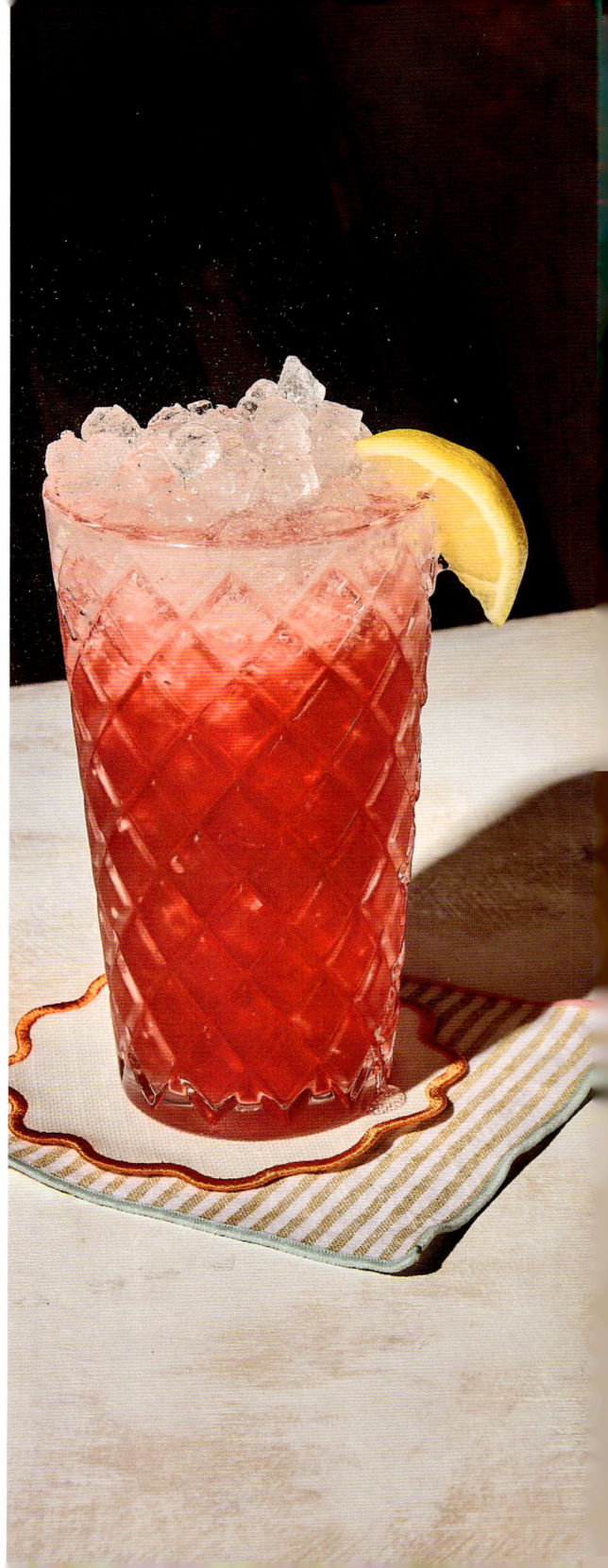

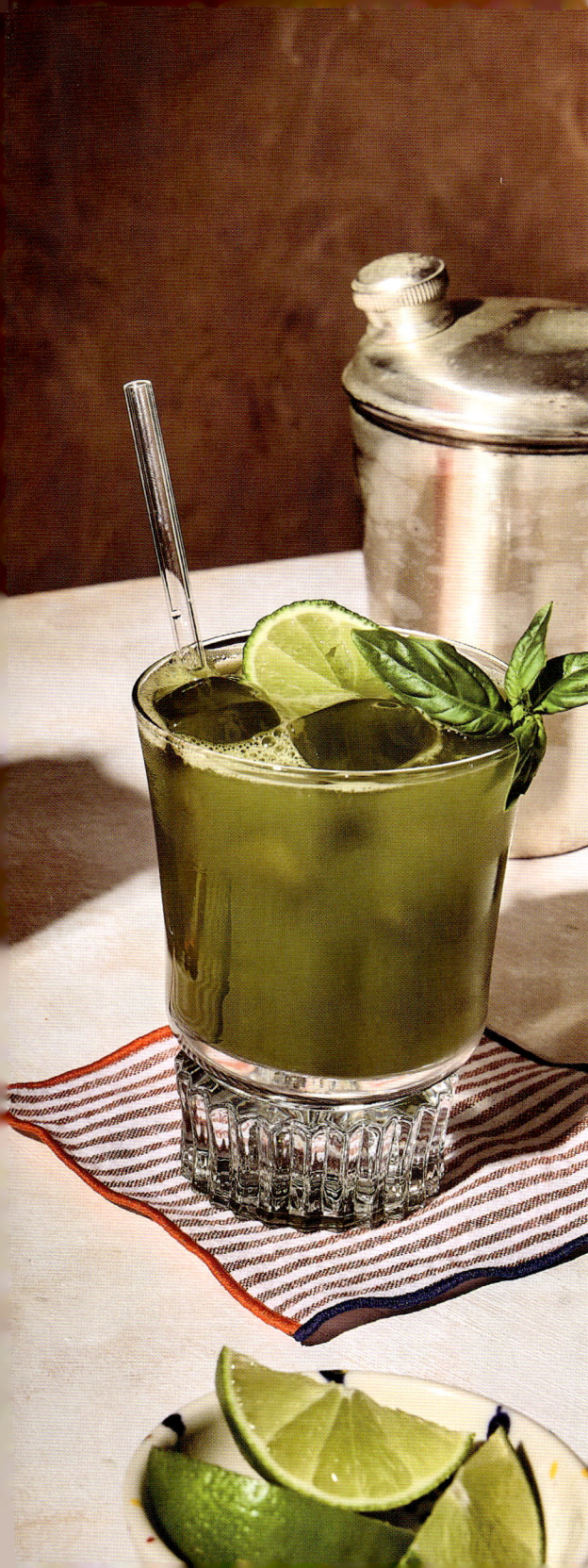

MATCHA BASIL LIMEADE

BASILINA
Buzz

SERVES 1

1 cup coconut water

Juice of 1 lime

2 basil leaves

½ teaspoon ceremonial-grade matcha powder

Ice cubes

GARNISH

1 lime wedge

1 basil leaf

1. Place the coconut water, lime juice, basil, and matcha powder in a blender. Blend until the basil leaves are broken down, about 20 seconds.

2. Fill a lowball glass with ice. Pour the blended mixture into the glass (strain through a fine-mesh sieve, if desired).

3. Stir and garnish with a lime wedge and a basil leaf.

Matcha and I have always had a complicated relationship: I want to love it, but not every sip wins me over. That's why Basilina Buzz was a total game changer for me. The earthy matcha blends effortlessly with the fresh basil and bright lime. The best part is how ridiculously easy it is to make, so even a matcha skeptic like myself can whip it up in no time. Trust me: This one's worth the buzz!

THE DETOX

SERVES 1

Juice of 1 lime

1 tablespoon agave syrup

½ teaspoon grated ginger (use ¼ teaspoon for less spice)

¼ teaspoon ground turmeric

Pinch of cayenne

1 cup coconut water, divided

Ice cubes

GARNISH

Candied ginger

Cayenne (optional)

1. Place the lime juice, agave, ginger, turmeric, and cayenne in a shaker and stir.

2. Add ½ cup coconut water and a handful of ice.

3. Shake until the outside of the shaker is frosty, about 5 seconds.

4. Fill a lowball glass with ice. Strain the juice mixture into the glass.

5. Add the remaining coconut water.

6. Garnish with candied ginger and an extra sprinkle of cayenne (if using).

Meet The Detox: a bold and spicy refresher that knows how to wake your taste buds and reset your vibe. With fiery ginger, a splash of citrus, and the right kick of spice, this drink is as invigorating as it is refreshing. It's time to detox from negative vibes, cleanse your mind, and embrace the positive energy around you.

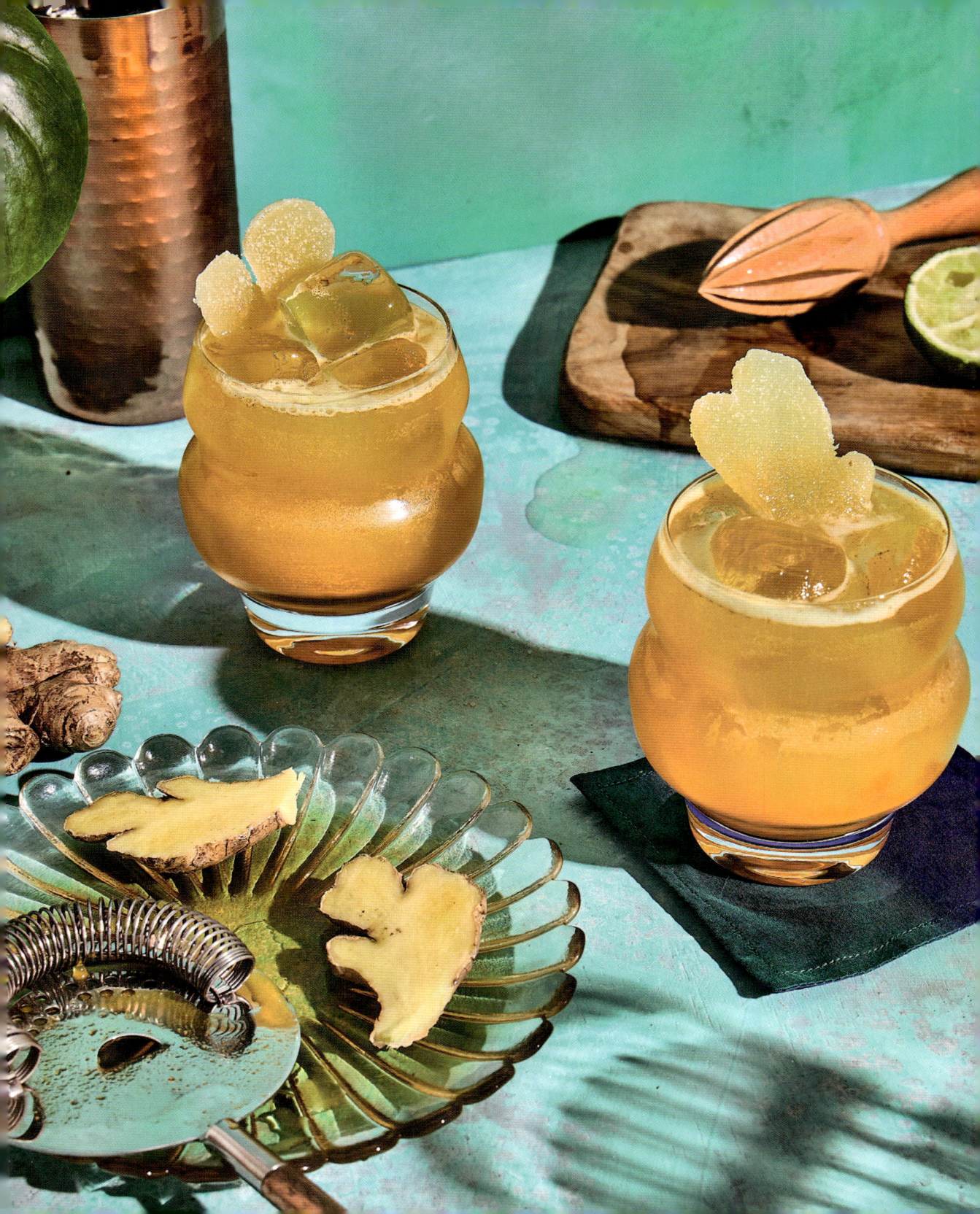

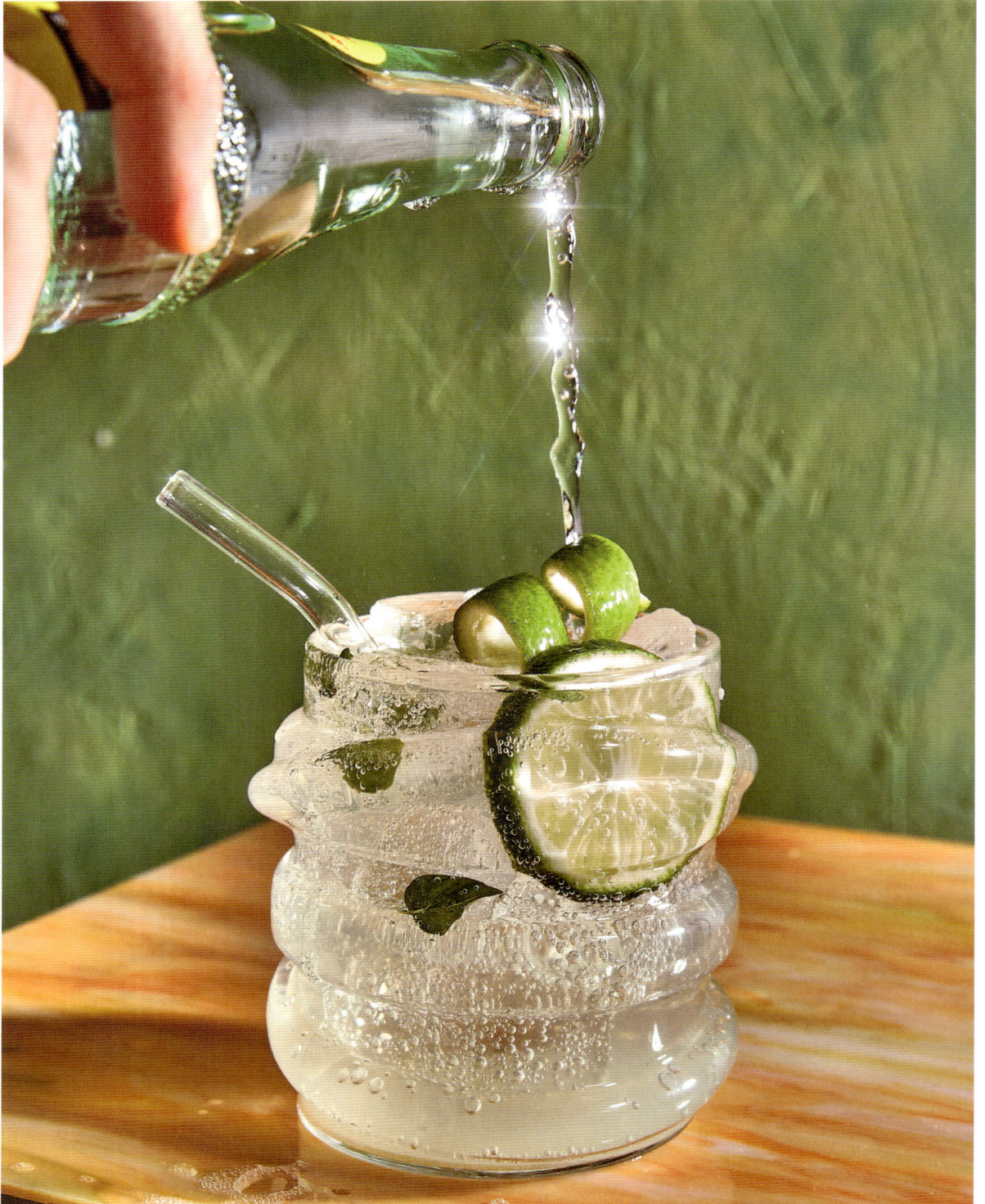

YUZU *AF*

SERVES 1

5 basil leaves

Juice of ½ lime

Ice cubes

1 cup yuzu sparkling water (I like Fever-Tree Sparkling Lime & Yuzu), chilled

GARNISH

Lime wheel

Basil leaves

1. Place the basil leaves and lime juice in a tall glass. Gently muddle with a muddler or the back of a wooden spoon to release the basil aroma, 4 to 5 twists.

2. Fill the glass with ice and top with sparkling water.

3. Stir and garnish with a lime wheel and basil leaves.

I was unfamiliar with yuzu until about a year ago, and wow, have I been missing out. Yuzu AF is bright, bold, and un-apologetically zesty, packing a punch of tart-sweetness in every sip. It is as refreshing as it is effortless, which is what makes it one of the quickest recipes in this book to whip up.

FROZEN COCOA SLUSH

FROSTY *Remix*

SERVES 1

1½ cups milk of choice, divided

½ avocado, diced

2 tablespoons agave syrup

1½ tablespoons cocoa powder

1 tablespoon nut butter (I use almond butter)

1 teaspoon vanilla extract

⅛ teaspoon salt

1. Pour ¾ cup milk into an ice cube tray and place in the freezer until completely frozen, about 3 hours (see Tip).

2. Place the milk ice cubes, remaining ¾ cup milk, avocado, agave, cocoa powder, nut butter, vanilla, and salt in a blender and blend until thick and whipped, 1 to 2 minutes.

3. Pour into a highball glass and enjoy.

TIP Don't add regular ice to this drink; it will water it down. Either make milk ice cubes in step 1 or make this drink without ice altogether (it will still be delicious, but the texture will be thinner).

FROZEN THIN MINT SLUSH
In the mood for a thin mint? Add 5 to 7 mint leaves to the blender in step 2 and enjoy.

PROTEIN FROSTY REMIX
Wanting more protein? Add ⅓ cup of your favorite protein powder.

I used to live for those chocolatey, brain-freezing, drive-thru frostys (honestly, I think I kept Wendy's in business). But this version? It's got all the creamy, cocoa goodness I loved, with less sugar and more balance (because, you know, adulthood). Grab a spoon or straw and take a delicious trip down memory lane.

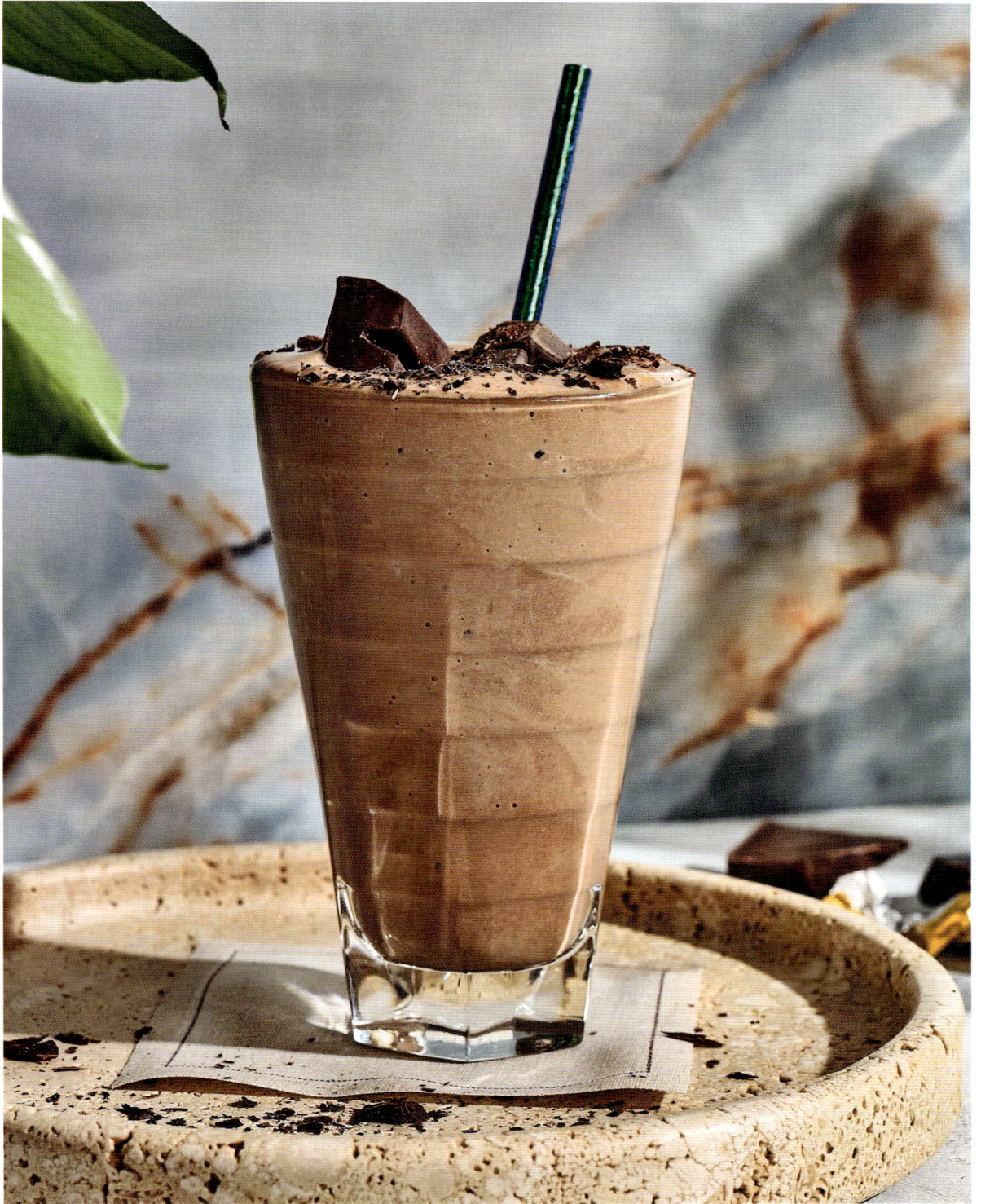

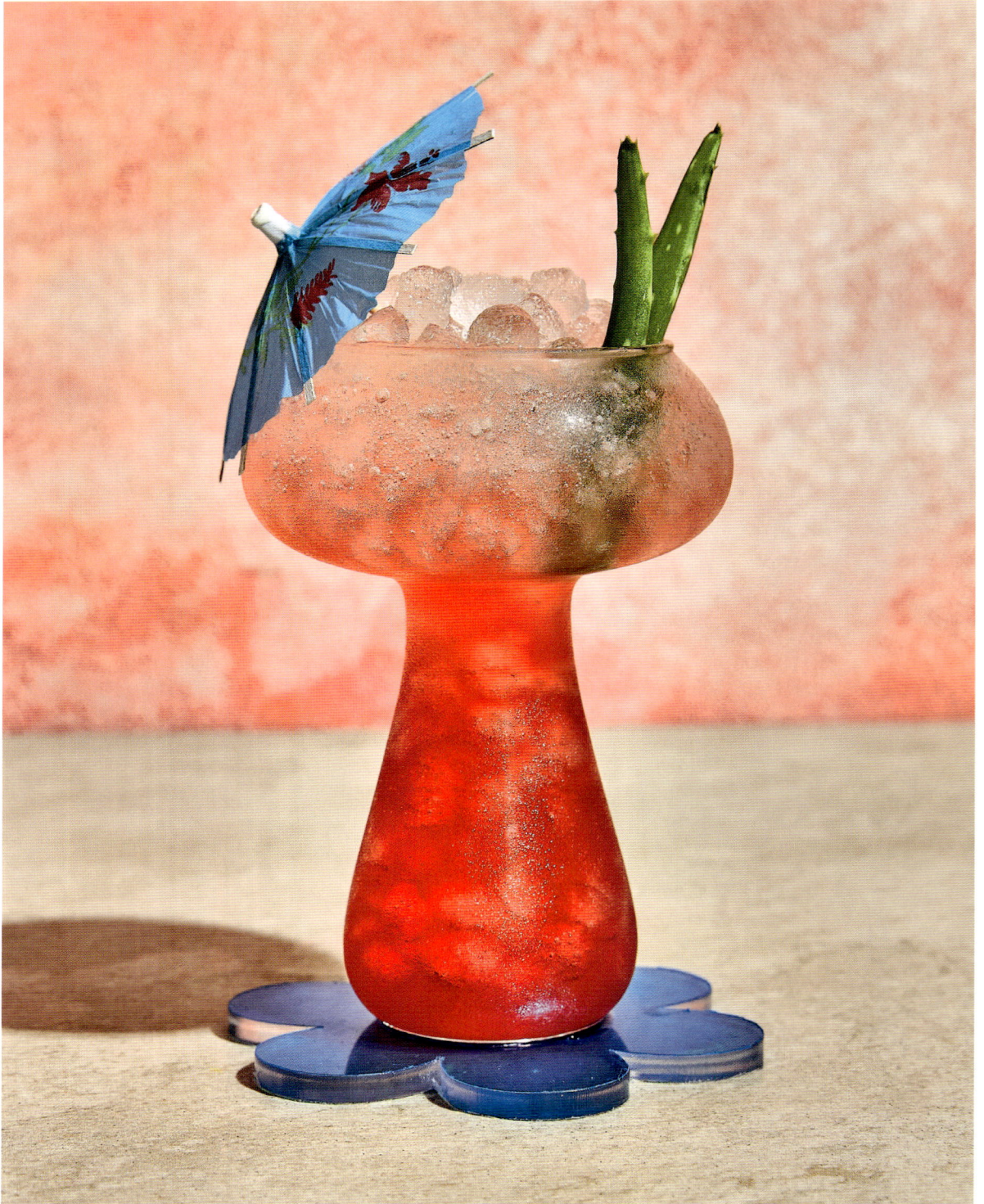

CONFIDENT *Cran*

SERVES 1

⅓ cup unsweetened cranberry juice

¼ cup aloe vera juice

Juice of ½ lemon

Ice cubes

¼ cup unflavored seltzer

1. Pour the cranberry juice, aloe vera juice, and lemon juice into a shaker and stir.

2. Add a handful of ice and shake until the outside of the shaker is frosty, about 5 seconds.

3. Fill a lowball glass with ice and strain in the chilled juice.

4. Top with seltzer and enjoy.

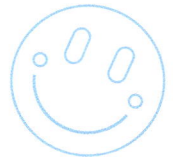

Say hello to Confident Cran, a mocktail that fuels your confidence and lets your inner glow shine. The aloe vera juice has many health benefits; full of powerful antioxidants, it's hydrating, gut-healthy, and great for your skin. When combined with the tart cranberry juice, it tastes like a Jolly Rancher—I kid you not.

Before & After a Workout

Go in with a plan: I love deciding what workout I'm going to do the night before or planning it in the morning while sipping my coffee. I feel it limits the procrastination time and allows me to get a move on with the least resistance.

Get the jams going: Music is motivation, and sometimes it's 2000s pop that brings me back to high school or feel-good country that feels like a warm summer night. Start playing those jams the moment you walk into the gym so you feel that energy from the get-go.

Warm that body up: Working out feels much better after a quick warm-up, for both the body and the mind. It's your time to truly focus on you and forget about outside stressors.

The brighter, the better: Pick out an outfit that makes you feel your best! On days I'm not feeling the greatest, throwing on bright colors immediately boosts my mood.

Rest and Recover: You can do all the workouts in the world but if you're not catching your zzz's, your muscles can't fully recover. Don't forget to hydrate before, during, and after (see the Sweat, Sip, Repeat chapter, starting on page 147).

Stretch it out: Don't forget to stretch—I know I do. As little as 5 minutes is better than nothing and can make a huge difference.

Don't overcomplicate it: One thing that keeps us from moving our bodies is taking it too seriously. Every workout doesn't have to be the hardest workout of your life. The goal is to create consistency with a routine that feels *good* for *you*.

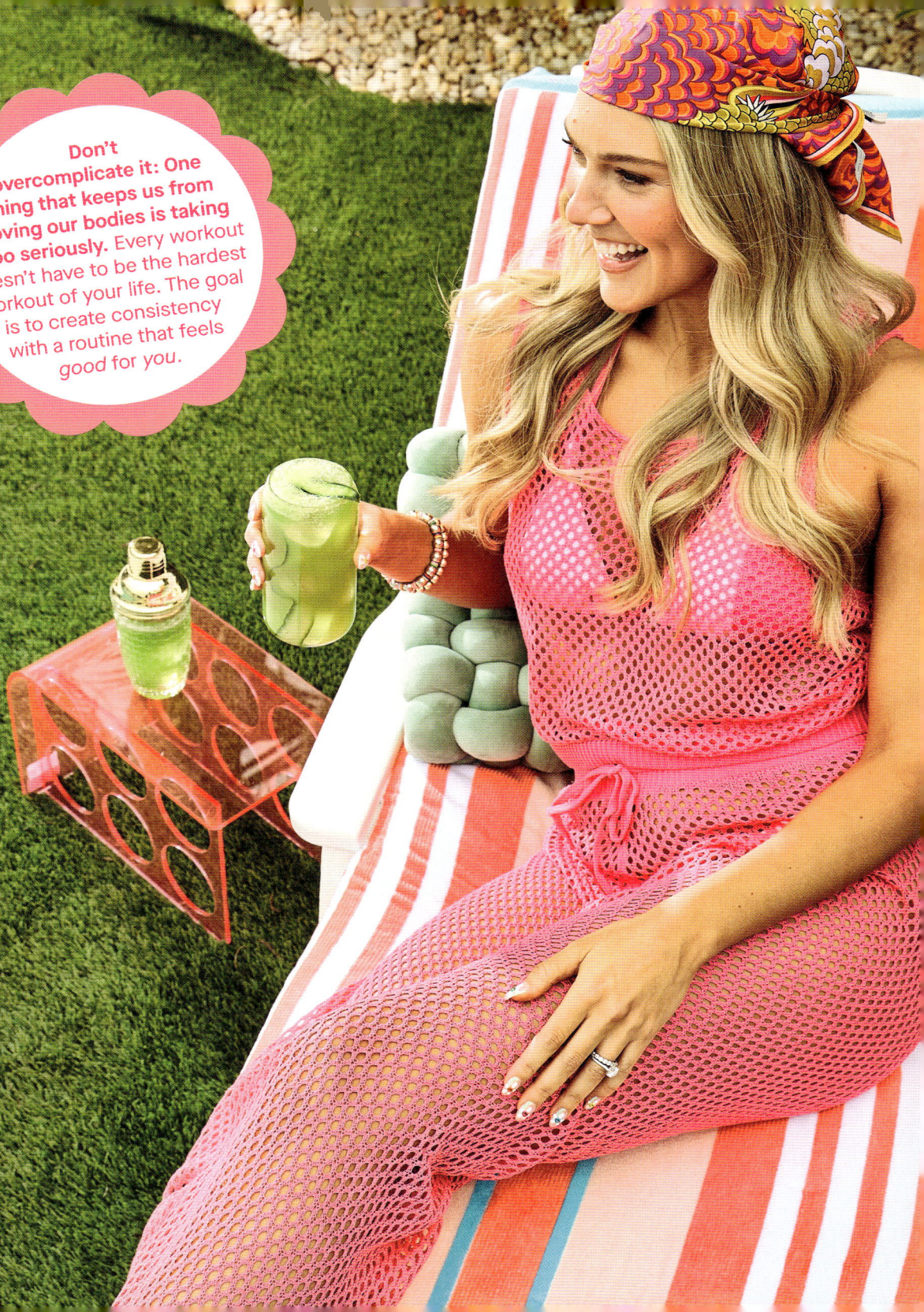

Index

ACKNOWLEDGMENTS

To be totally honest, writing a book was never on my radar. Not because I didn't want to do it, but because it always seemed like a far-off dream—something so out of reach that I never really allowed myself to imagine it as part of my future. But then Amanda, my literary agent, noticed my passion for mocktails and reached out to suggest I write a mocktail book. So, huge thank you to Amanda for seeing something in me that I didn't even see in myself.

Working with Amanda led me to Olivia, my amazing editor, who was just as passionate about this book as I was. She believed in my vision from day one, and I'm forever grateful for her time, effort, and enthusiasm in making this book a reality. I still can't believe I'm with the #1 publisher—it feels so surreal! Olivia, you're the reason I believe dreams can evolve, because you helped me create a whole new dream that I never thought possible. Big shout-out to the entire DK team for all the work put into this project. I am so grateful!

To my husband, Chris, thank you for being my rock. From taste-testing every single mocktail (yes, even the weird ones!) to reminding me that I could do this while pregnant and navigating new motherhood, your support means the world to me. I love you endlessly, and I couldn't have done this without you.

To my parents, thank you for trusting me and my unique path since I was little. I can only imagine the questions you had about where my career was going to go, and believe me, I didn't see a book coming either! But I have always followed my gut, and you didn't ask questions. I'm so grateful for that. And, of course, thank you for all the times you watched your grandson so I could work on this book!

To Karen and Tom, my in-laws, thank you for being part of this journey. From picking up ingredients to giving me honest feedback, you helped shape this book into something I'm truly proud of.

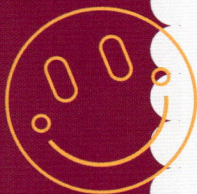

To my management team—thank you for always having my back and pouring into all facets of my life. Your hard work, belief in me, and constant support have made all the difference in bringing this to life. Thank you for pushing me to go after all the things I want to pursue. I couldn't ask for a better team by my side.

To Ashleigh, the photographer of my dreams, thank you, thank you, thank you. This book would not be what it is without you. You are a gem!

To Amy, the incredible designer of this book, who made it beautiful and bright—just how I like it. Your talent is incredible, and I'm grateful for it!

A special thank you to my friend Holland, my stylist for the photo shoot, and Gabriella, my hair and makeup queen. You made me feel fabulous.

And, of course, to my amazing community, whether you're here for the workouts, the Charly content, or the Trader Joe's obsession, your unwavering support helps me show up as my true self every day. I want this book to serve as a tool for you to do the same, because we all deserve to feel our best and to feel confident in choosing to do so. This book is for you, and I hope you love it as much as I do.

Cheers to having the courage and confidence to believe in ourselves, to prioritize self-care, and to always choose to bring our own energy.

Thank you all from the bottom of my heart!

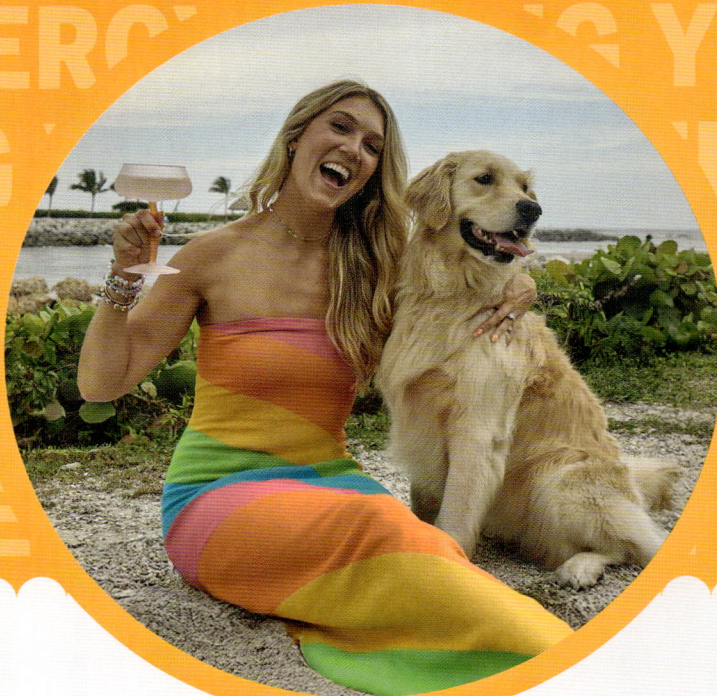

About the Author

Callie Gullickson is a human mom, dog mom, wife, Peloton instructor, Lululemon ambassador, Florida native, and creator of healthy, attainable, and balanced routines. Known as your sunshine BFF, she inspires people to have confidence in their everyday lives and embrace what makes them unique! She encourages people to move their body, make mindful choices, and have fun along the way. Callie is known for her positive outlook, reminding others to always BYOE: bring your own energy.

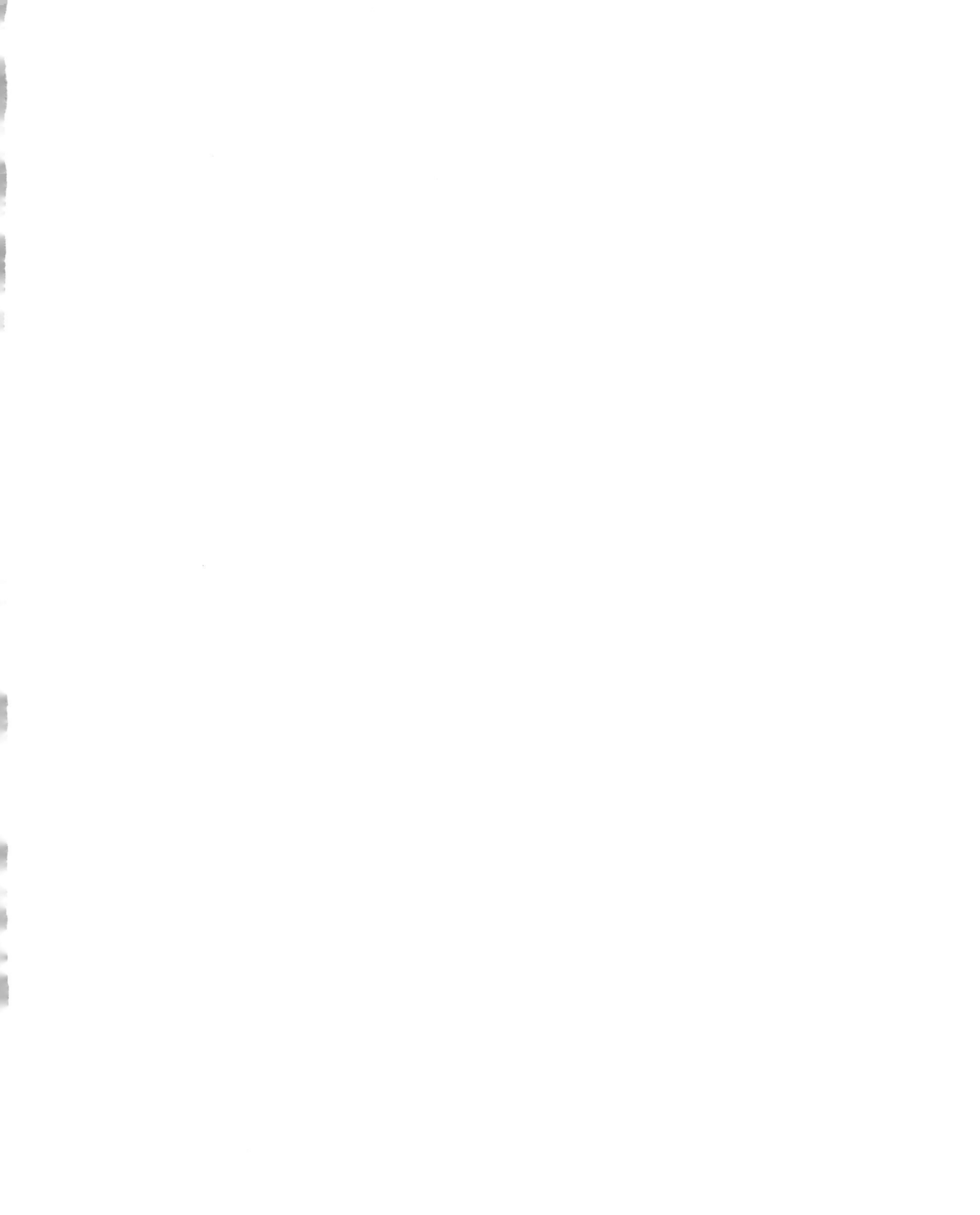